For many years, Dr Maureen Corrigan was a medical practitioner who worked in a broad range of healthcare roles, from general practitioner to CEO. She retired early as a result of developing multiple sclerosis (MS). Maureen is now able to pursue her many other passions, including travel and writing, which has led her to say, 'I sometimes think getting MS was the best thing that happened to me!'

MAUREEN T. CORRIGAN

UNEXPECTED REWARDS

TRAVELLING TO THE ARCTIC WITH A MOBILITY SCOOTER

Published by Vivid Publishing
P.O. Box 948, Fremantle
Western Australia 6959
www.vividpublishing.com.au

National Library of Australia Cataloguing-in-Publication data:
Creator: Corrigan, Maureen T., author.
Title: Unexpected Rewards : travelling to the Arctic with a mobility scooter / Maureen T. Corrigan.
ISBN: 9781925442472 (paperback)
Subjects: Corrigan, Maureen T.--Travel.
Multiple sclerosis--Patients--Biography.
People with disabilities--Travel--Norway.
People with disabilities--Travel--Arctic regions.
People with disabilities--Life skills guides.
Norway--Description and travel.
Arctic regions--Description and travel.
Dewey Number: 910.873

This book is dedicated to

Noeleen P. Corrigan
My mother – who gave me the travel bug
as well as a string of lessons for life

and

Jan Stow
A valued friend who motivated me to write this book.

ACKNOWLEDGEMENTS

Vaarunika Dharmapala, my editor, for her invaluable assistance, direction and work. Jane Mundy, a friend and writer, for her encouragement, support, and readiness to bounce ideas around. Yasmin Gray, from Fontaine Publishing Group for her patience and help with publishing.

CONTENTS

PART ONE:

IN THE LEAD-UP

CHAPTER 1

A NEW LIFE

I've always loved travelling, especially to places with a bit of an edge to them. Some of those places have been very exciting and I always wanted more. But in recent years, the way I travel has changed dramatically. I have trouble walking and I need mobility aids; this is because I developed multiple sclerosis (MS).

So many things have happened to me while I've been travelling with walking aids – so many funny things. My aids have ended up giving me more interesting and funny stories to tell than when I travelled without them!

With that change, I thought I had to do a lot more planning and checking before I left on a trip in order to feel confident, so I'd know what to expect and be prepared. Well, I *was* a Queen's Guide! I was taught the Girl Guide motto 'Be Prepared'. I still have my shirt with its badges (I loved getting those badges!), and the motto is still inside me.

As well as some form of aid, I also need someone to go travelling with. I can't manage the devices on my own. Nor can I carry a bag of clothes and whatever else I need and ride my scooter at the same time.

Luckily, I have a wonderful friend who is my flatmate and who also loves travelling. Sue, who is just a bit older than me, is fit, able and happy to help.

I first met Sue when we worked together at a university hospital in the late 1970s – a long time ago. We've been friends ever since, and our paths crossed at different times, sometimes with many years in between. We've always got along well and our friendship has got better as we got older.

Sue is her own person and we make a great team. Our skills and interests complement each other. We can chat easily or be silent. She's great company and we have a lot of laughs.

I may have had MS for just over twenty years, but it wasn't until 2006 that I was diagnosed with secondary progressive MS. That's serious stuff.

What is MS? Good, reliable, up-to-date information can be found on various websites, such as those produced by MS Australia, the MS Society in the UK, the National MS Society in the US and the MS International Federation.

Very simply, MS is an autoimmune disease that causes the body to reject and destroy the myelin conducting fibres of nerves in the central nervous system – that is, the brain and spinal cord. The transmission of information becomes slowed, interrupted or stopped. The cause of MS is unknown and there is no cure.

The main physical symptoms of MS are problems with mobility, bladder and bowel functions, vision, speech and fatigue. Mobility and fatigue are my main problems, with a bit of bladder thrown in.

Everyone with MS has different symptoms, and we're all at different stages and rates of progression. We also have something in common, but there's a great range in how severe each person's problems are.

New treatments are changing what happens in the course of the disease, and I believe it's important to keep up to date with a good neurologist who has an interest in MS. I receive four-weekly infusions of a monoclonal antibody type of drug called Tysabri (Natalizumab).

Early in my diagnosis, I read that MS was characterised as a disease that causes slowly progressive paralysis. One of my first thoughts was that at least it was slower than motor neurone disease (MND). That was a terrible disease.

My employment background is in health – in management, administration and the corporate side of hospitals and health services. I started my university education with a bachelor of science degree but changed to medicine when it hit me that being a doctor was the only thing I wanted. I ended up with a medical degree from the University of Sydney, a masters in health administration from the University of NSW and a college fellowship in medical administration. I was very proud of what added up to ten years at university. I spent the early years after graduation as a general practitioner, but I loved being where I ended up. At the time I was diagnosed, my career was still progressing.

When I realised that I couldn't continue to work as the CEO of a large organisation, my first reaction was incredible disappointment. I loved working. We'd just finished the first stage of a massive change management programme and it was an exciting time. There was more to do. Suddenly, I had to stop and think about a new life. I'd wanted and expected to be working well into my sixties or seventies, but I had to stop at the youthful age of fifty-three.

My next response was to just deal with it the best I could.

I finally found the best neurologist I could and followed his advice and recommended treatments. I also tried to learn as much as I could about MS. I'd never encountered it closely before. I joined the MS Society, received their newsletters and went to their information sessions. I saw a physiotherapist and did exercise programmes. I rested every day. I tried to eat a healthy, balanced diet. What else could I do?

Being located in Melbourne wasn't essential any more. Where was the best place to live with my MS? I'd worked and lived in all four of the states on the eastern side of Australia – Queensland, NSW, Victoria and Tasmania. I was familiar with all of them. I'd bought a house in Queensland some years back, but had been working and living in Melbourne in more recent years. With my MS, for most of the year Queensland was too hot and humid for me. Melbourne was cooler most of the time; it was also flat, easy to get around and it had a highly accessible public transport system.

I decided that Melbourne would be my new home base for the foreseeable future.

For the first time, I needed help with daily living. Sue had recently retired, after thirty-five years of working and helping other people. Now she became my carer. Melbourne, with its famous sandbelt of golf courses, was also the perfect place for her, with her passion for golf.

It occurred to me fairly quickly that because I wasn't working any more I had a lot of free time. Some time was taken up with medical appointments, infusions, exercise and rest. But I could see I'd have time available to do the things I loved, especially travelling.

I accepted the fact that I had MS and tried to find ways around it. What was I able to do with my current abilities? My right hand wasn't affected, and I had to sit a lot of the time. I could see, talk and think. Writing, reading and more travelling were my first picks. I also took a greater interest in managing my financial affairs, as well as playing the stock market and trading.

Having MS was a new phase in my life, an opportunity. I've always had a very positive attitude – I've been called 'Pollyanna' more than once in the past! I can still hear my mother's voice saying, 'Where there's a will, there's a way'. She was always encouraging and she was very proud of me. 'You can do anything you want to,' she said, and I believed her.

There had to be ways around difficulties. Anything was possible, you just had to organise it. I was a good organiser. But organising my reduced mobility was going to be one of the most interesting challenges I'd faced so far.

I caught the travel bug from my mother, and I loved it for so many reasons. I loved learning, seeing and experiencing something new. I found everything involved with travelling to be exciting. But for the trip I was planning in 2011, I felt I had to approach it in a different way.

PART TWO:

PLANNING

CHAPTER 1
THE IDEA

Going on the trip to Norway and the Arctic was very important to me. But why go to those places? How did I arrive at that choice? I think the idea came about because of the polar bears. I wanted to see them in their natural habitat. I was sure Sue would want to see them even more than I did. She has a special feeling for animals and wildlife. As my friend and carer, it was important that she was happy with the trip. We always travelled together these days.

I also wanted to go to a place that was unusual, somewhere far away, with some remoteness – a place that had a bit of an edge to it, somewhere that had some extra excitement going for it.

Gwen, who lives in the same apartment block as Sue and me, had spoken to us about a trip she'd been on a few years earlier. She'd told us that her trip had circumnavigated the island of Spitsbergen in the Arctic. We must have been talking about wonderful animals, starting with her dog and then somehow moving on to polar bears. Gwen had a beautiful dog called Lilly, a Sheltie – a miniature Lassie dog – who, like the bears, had some long white fur!

Her trip sounded wonderful, and when we joined her for a drink one day Gwen brought out some photos. 'You might like to have a look at these. They were taken from the ship, we were so close.' They were very good photos of polar bears. I hadn't planned our yearly overseas trip yet and, yes, it was then that the seed was planted.

We'd also recently watched a television programme, a Global Village series, on one of the SBS channels. It showed Geirangerfjord in Norway. The scenery was stunning. That place became etched on my brain to see one day for sure.

I hadn't been to any Scandinavian countries before. Sue had been in the early 1970s. She'd travelled around most of Europe then, from her working base in London. However, she hadn't been further north in Norway than Trondheim. A trip further north would therefore include new territory for both of us. That was yet another reason to go to the Arctic area.

The Northern Lights came up at some stage. Unfortunately, I realised after a few enquiries that the polar bears came out in the northern summer and the lights were best in the northern winter. However, the lights were always there, and the darker the sky and the fewer the clouds, the easier it was to see them. If we were lucky, we might be able to see the lights anyway.

Yes, that's how I decided in 2010 to start looking in more detail about going to Norway and the Svalbard Arctic region for next year's overseas trip. How would we go there?

I recalled hearing a few years ago about the Hurtigruten coastal run in Norway. But I wanted to go further north than the coast of Norway to be able to see the polar bears. The bears lived on the island of Spitsbergen in the Svalbard region, not on the mainland of Norway. The island was about one thousand kilometres to the north-west, well away from the coast of Norway.

There were boat trips like Gwen's advertised, ones that went only around the island, and there were separate trips that covered the mainland coastal route of Norway. I wanted to go to both areas. When I did see trips advertised going to the two places, they involved flying between two different boat trips. The other thing I wanted was to stay on board the same boat. I didn't want to pack and unpack or negotiate any more airports than I needed to. It was more difficult for me at airports these days, with my mobility problems and aids.

The type of ship that we'd take was important too. I wanted to get off the ship to be in the natural environment. I had in mind something like the inflatable boats – Zodiacs, they were called – that we took on our Antarctic trip in January 2008. Those small, ten-person vessels brought you so close to wildlife and nature. It was wonderful to be on one. And, like Antarctica, we both wanted to be on more of an expedition than a cruise.

We didn't want to dress up formally at night or be entertained with shows. However, we did want to listen to talks and lectures by professionals, about the area we were travelling in and the wildlife living there. The ship also had to have a lift (important for my gear) and be accessible for me. There shouldn't be too many passengers either – not a number in the thousands. About two hundred would be plenty.

When I saw a brochure advertising an expedition cruise trip commencing in Longyearbyen, the capital of the Svalbard region, after a flight from Oslo, I was very excited. The route on the rough map provided spoke to me. I took a photo of the map on the brochure so I could refer back to it as I planned the trip. (Photo 2.1.1)

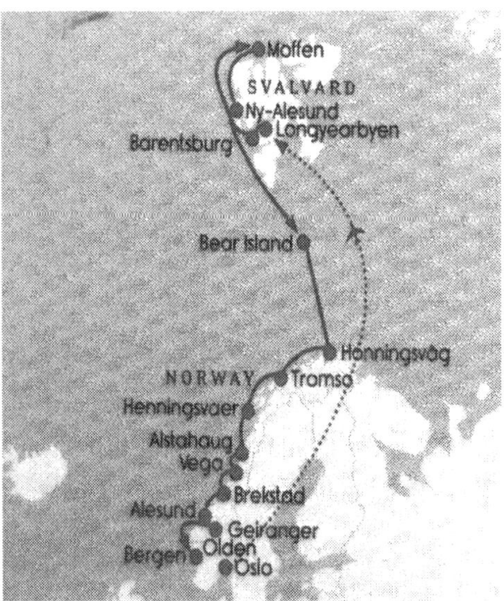

Photo 2.1.1 Map of our expedition cruise
Image credit: Hurtigruten

The ship was the MS *Fram*. It was a special Hurtigruten ship and usually went on voyages around Iceland, Greenland and the Svalbard region in the northern summer, and to Antarctica in the southern summer. The trip was apparently a new schedule that included parts of the coast of Norway after leaving Svalbard on its way south to Antarctica. The passenger capacity was about two hundred to three hundred. I thought it looked like a fine ship for our cruise. (Photo 2.1.2)

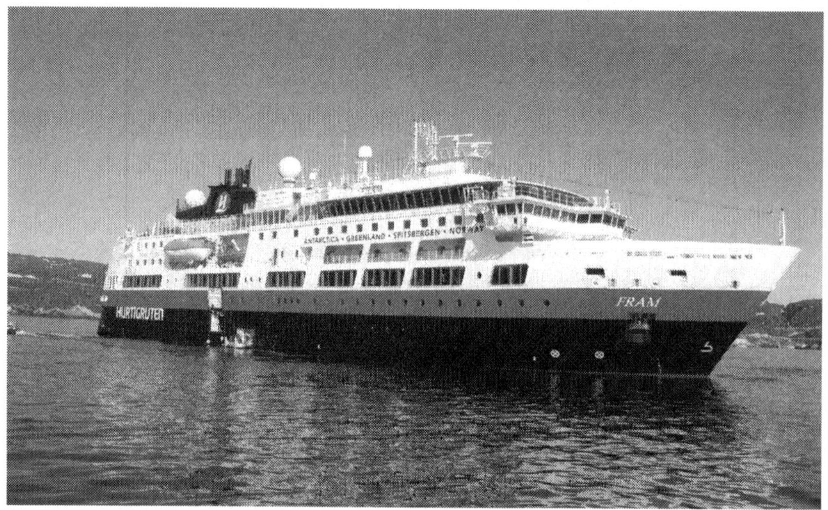

Photo 2.1.2 The MS *Fram*

The MS *Fram* was used for expedition trips, or what were advertised as 'explorer voyages'. The ship had craft on board called polar circle boats. The photos in the advertising material showed these as light metal craft, with outboard motors. They could take about ten people. They had steps to board and disembark, and a rail down the middle to hold. That looked even better for me than the Zodiacs. I can walk short distances and get up and down a few steps very slowly. I thought those boats should work out okay for me.

There was only one trip advertised. It was in September of the following year, 2011. That was at the end of the polar bear season and there was also the possibility of seeing the Northern Lights.

The ship had a lift and there were no formal evenings. It was an expedition cruise, with talks and lectures by naturalists and other scientists. It all seemed ideal.

Whenever I decided to travel, I'd think of my mother. She was in her eighties at the time and had a passion for travelling. She'd already travelled to many places in the world but still loved going away.

Mum had been to Norway on an excursion from England many years ago. It had been a short trip of a few days to see some fjords and the city of Bergen. She still had the article advertising the trip filed away after nearly thirty years. Mum also kept postcards as souvenirs. I kept a lot too. She'd sent one to me from Norway and I'd had to give it back! She sent both of those items to me in the mail when I said I was thinking of travelling to Norway.

The scene on the front of her postcard was of Geirangerfjord with two ships in the water. Someone was sitting on the edge of a mountain overlooking a town and the fjord. (Photo 2.1.3)

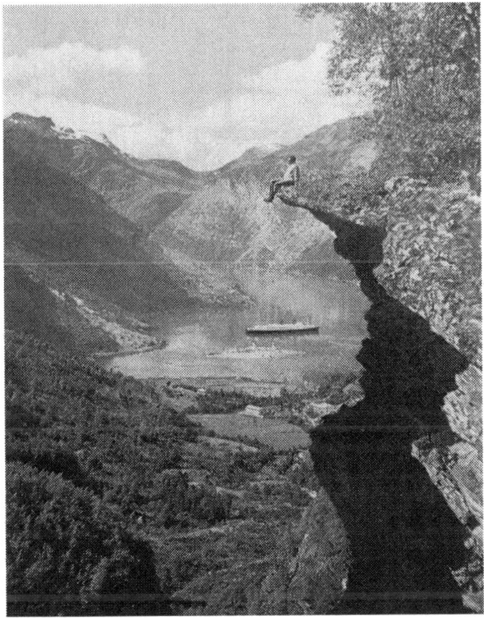

Photo 2.1.3 Mum's postcard of Geirangerfjord
Image credit: Photo Normanns Kunstforlag

Printed on the back was 'Norway: Flydalsjuvet abyss Geiranger. Foto: Normann. T-13-66'. It was an excellent picture.

Stamped on the back of the postcard was the postmark of Bergen with the date '11–9.84'. Mum's writing on the card had the date at the top of '9.9.84'. (Photo 2.1.4)

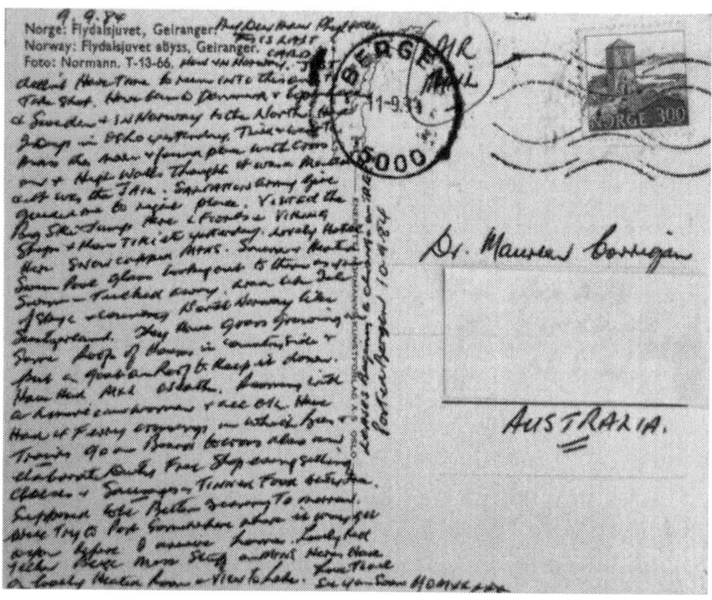

Photo 2.1.4 Back of Mum's postcard

Mum's writing on her postcards was a little difficult to read but there was always something humorous in them. Her use of upper and lower cases was also interesting. My interpretation of her writing, exactly as it was set out on the card is here:

> My dear Maur Phil & Den
> This is LAST
> CARD.
> Now IN Norway JUST
> didn't Have Time to run INTO this one to
> Take shot. Have been to Denmark & Copenhagen
> & Sweden & iN Norway to the North. Had

> 2 Days in Oslo yesterday. Tried & went to
> Mass this morn & found place with cross
> on & High Walls thought it was a Monastery
> & it was the JAIL. SALVATION army girl
> guided me to right place. Visited the
> Big Ski Jump Here & Fiords & Viking
> Ships & Kon TIKI yesterday. Lovely Hotel
> Here SNOW capped MtNS. Sauna & Heated
> Swim Pool glass looking out to them as if your
> Swimming Tucked away. area like Isle
> of Skye & country North Norway like
> Switzerland. They have grass growing on
> Some Roofs of Houses in countryside &
> put a goat on Roof to Keep it down.
> Have Had Mxd weather. Rooming with
> a American woman & all OK. Have
> Heard of Ferry crossings in which Bus &
> Trains go on Board to cross also an
> elaborate Duty Free Shop even selling
> cheeses & Sausages & TINNed Food Duty Free.
> Supposed to be Better Scenery Tomorrow.
> Will Try to Post Somewhere where it may get
> to you Before I arrive home. Lovely Red
> Yellow Beige Moss Stuff on MTNS Here Have
> a lovely Heated Room & View to Lake.
> Love To all
> See you Soon MOM xxxxx

There was more writing up the middle at right angles:

> Leaves Beginning to change on TREES
> Posted Bergen 10.9.84

Mum had come to Egypt and Jordan with us in January 2010. My brother Dennis and his wife Paddy came to help me, but Mum was the one who'd ended up needing more help to get around than we'd anticipated. She had trouble walking, which was unusual for her. Not long after arriving back home, she'd improved.

When we went to Antarctica with her, two years earlier in January 2008, she was fine. She didn't need any help and loved it. I thought she might be interested in coming to Norway and the Arctic with us next year if she felt up to it.

Dennis was not on the Antarctic trip, but the polar regions fascinated him. He might be interested in coming on a trip to the Arctic with us. It would be to help Mum mostly, in case she needed him again. He would also be a good backup for me. Dennis was big, strong and very thoughtful.

When Christmastime 2010 came around, I saw a special deal on the internet for the trip that I had in mind. There was ten per cent off if you booked and paid a deposit by the end of December. Mum was having Christmas with Dennis that year. He lived in Ballina, in northern NSW, and so there were many STD phone calls racked up over that season.

After a lot of discussion about the ship, the cabins, deck levels, the beds, the possibility of seasickness, the number of airport transfers and similar concerns, Mum decided that yes, it was worth it, she'd come. Dennis said yes too. He'd come on his own and share a cabin with her.

In late December 2010, I booked the Hurtigruten trip – for four people and two cabins – through a travel agent, just in time for the discount.

Some weeks later, when Mum was back at her home on the NSW Central Coast, she rang me and left a message. 'Oh, it's just Mum here, love. Nothing urgent. I'll call you back later. It's … ah … about 9.30 on Monday. I just wanted to have a chat with you about something. I'll ring you back later. Thank you, love. Thank you. Mum here. I'll call you later.'

When I talked with her soon afterwards, she said, 'My back's not too good, love. I don't think I can go on the trip with you. Will you be all right on your own?'

Dennis was really going for Mum's sake. He would also have helped me too, I'm sure. In Egypt, he carried me on his back to get down and back up the long flights of steps to the River Nile. We went on a felucca ride in Aswan and had to get from road level down to the boat on the water at low tide. It was a long way down. Mum managed those steps then, even though she had trouble walking. But now she was older and frailer.

After many more conversations, I cancelled the booking for the two of them. That left Sue and me. I realised then that since my diagnosis of MS, Sue and I hadn't travelled outside Australia alone. My mobility aids had to be loaded and unloaded into cars, buses and planes. Sue had always had help before. We discussed whether we'd manage, and decided we would. We kept our booking.

The expedition cruise that I'd booked was called 'Polar Bears, Islands and Fjords'. It started in Oslo in the south-east of Norway and finished in Bergen thirteen days later on Norway's south-west coast. There were set dates and arrangements for the cruise package, starting with a flight leaving Oslo on 7 September and finishing with the ship arriving in Bergen on 19 September. I had to plan and book the rest of the trip.

I got out my 2011 calendar, photocopied the month of September and wrote on it all the dates for my infusions at the hospital. Because I had intravenous Tysabri every four weeks, I had to arrange travelling around those dates.

I could change the infusion day by about a week or two, but not more than that and not very often. I highlighted and marked the dates of the cruise on my calendar and took note of all the infusion dates in and around September. It looked like I'd have to change one date by two weeks. I thought I'd double-check that with my neurologist.

I bought the *Lonely Planet Norway* guide, looked at websites and did some reading. I also spoke with people I knew who loved travelling for ideas about Norway.

My next immediate job was to get us to Oslo and then back home to Melbourne. I wanted to work out the best way to fly to Oslo and exactly when we'd leave and come back, fitting it in around my infusions. Flying from Australia to Europe was such a distance that I thought I'd try to make the flight interesting but not too tiring.

I spent time viewing several airline websites. I looked at times, routes and prices. The price didn't matter that much as they were all about the same. Sue and I always flew economy class. We didn't need extra room and the service was good enough. We couldn't see the benefit of the higher cost. Everyone likes to get a good deal, so I kept a lookout for specials as well.

Trying to get to Oslo with a minimum of changes seemed to be challenging. If we did have a stopover, where would that be? It would have to be somewhere that was easy, interesting and not too hot. My first look had planes changing at Heathrow – no. Then there was Frankfurt – no. So big, I thought. What about a smaller European airport? That was another line of thinking. Then I thought about getting there via Dubai, Bangkok, Hong Kong or a Japanese city.

That January, I was on the phone to my friend Carolyn in Brisbane more often than usual. There were terrible floods up there. The Brisbane River had broken its banks. The river was flooding into the city and low-lying suburbs. The events were on the news every day. A monsoon trough was moving over northern Australia and the rains had been extra-heavy that year. Carolyn lived near the top of a very big hill, so she was safe. But she still couldn't get out and go too far for a while.

One day, when I was talking with Carolyn, she mentioned her upcoming travel plans. She and some friends in Brisbane were going on a trip to Norway, including a cruise. I was astounded. They were some of our best friends and I hadn't heard of their trip. 'Really?' I said.

'Yes, why?' said Carolyn.

'I've just booked a cruise in Norway!'

'You're joking!'

'No, I'm not. When are you going?'

'We're going on the Norway part of the trip on 8 June.'

They were going on the Hurtigruten coastal voyage – the old Norwegian coast postal run – three months before our planned trip. They were starting in Oslo and going overland to Bergen to board the ship. From Bergen, they were sailing north up the coast to near the Russian border. Then they'd fly back south from the town of Kirkenes. They'd be back in Brisbane on 5 July, about two months before we were due to leave.

Carolyn was flying from Brisbane to Düsseldorf via Dubai, and then going to Oslo from there. They were breaking the trip at Düsseldorf to stay in Germany for a while. Düsseldorf was yet another stop for us to consider. There were direct flights from there to Oslo, and Carolyn said it was a small and manageable airport.

That conversation with Carolyn about travelling to Norway was the first of many. She also ended up doing a reconnaissance for us, to check a side trip called 'Norway in a Nutshell', which I'll explain later.

After weeks of searching and thinking, the flights to Oslo still didn't gel with me. There seemed to be too many connections and the time it took to get there seemed longer than it needed to be. I didn't like any of the suggestions that came from the travel agent who did our cruise booking. They just didn't feel right.

In the middle of these days of beginning to plan and book a trip to Norway, I also had to have a routine magnetic resonance imaging (MRI) scan of my brain. I had it on 8 February. It was my fourth one and the result was good news. The lesions in my brain were unchanged since my last MRI, and there were no new ones forming. This took my attention away from thinking about our flight route for just a little while.

Then I remembered that there was another travel agent I could try. A friend had recommended a particular agency in the past. Even though my first contact with them for information about another trip had been a disaster, I thought I'd try them again. The person I'd dealt with before was away when I phoned. The new person who returned my call was very helpful and quickly pointed out that there was a direct flight to Oslo from Bangkok departing from Melbourne with Thai Airways. It was available for travel in the month of September and was on special. Decision made.

Booking that flight meant that certain other bookings also had to be made. I needed wheelchair assistance as usual, but what was different for the Norway and Arctic trip was my new scooter. I'd never travelled overseas with it before, and it had to be booked in as well.

***

I'll always remember going to my first MS Society information day. It was for people who had recently been diagnosed, and I was afraid of going. I was afraid of what I might see there. I asked Sue to come with me, but I walked into the meeting without any aids and without any help at all.

After a little while, I couldn't help but look around – I tried to be very subtle – to see what other people looked like. I wanted to see what might be in store for me in the future. So I studied them. Everyone looked as if there was absolutely nothing wrong with them at all! Just like me. No one was in a wheelchair, but there were plenty of questions about wheelchairs when it came to question time.

There were a few men in the audience but it was mostly women. MS is known to affect three times as many women as men. Most people at the session seemed to be aged in their twenties or thirties. That fitted the statistics as well. But I was older than that, and I found out why much later.

Many years ago, I'd thought about what I might do if I ended up in a wheelchair for some reason, such as an accident. I love sport so I'd thought, Oh well, I'll just become a wheelchair athlete. I'll enter competitions and be in the Paralympics. It didn't occur to me that I'd need strength in my upper body and arms, as well as stamina, to roll a wheelchair along, let alone compete in races.

Not long after that MS meeting, a mobility scooter was recommended to me.

I'll also always remember going to the Independent Living Centre (ILC) in Footscray, to meet up with an occupational therapist and test out several scooters for the first time. I didn't enjoy riding any of them. They were too big and bulky, and just looked and felt too obvious. I didn't feel like myself. It wasn't me who was riding them!

I tried to convince myself that I didn't really need one. I could still drive and my right leg was okay. I'd just drive right up to where I wanted to go and walk the very short distance to get wherever it was that I was going. But I did need something. Some distances were just too far to walk.

The best way to get around this, I decided, was to get a small movable chair – a 'Go Chair', it was called. It was red, and I could break it up into four small pieces and put it in the boot of my car. I could also use it at my desk at home. It worked out well for a while.

That seems a long time ago, but it wasn't really, only a few years. I've become much more pragmatic and accepting since then. I need aids so I can walk, and that's all there is to it. So I bought aids and I used them.

In October 2010, I once again went to the ILC. I was always looking for better, easier, lighter devices, especially for travelling. I kept an eye out all the time. The ILC had a lot of good information and a showroom of hundreds of disability products and devices. While there, I saw a video of a new scooter, just out, called a 'Luggie'. As soon as I saw it, I wanted it. It looked fantastic.

Within a few days, I was the proud owner of a bright new Luggie scooter. It was easy to collapse, and easy for a helper to wheel and load. It had a light, two-kilogram lithium battery that lasted a long time, and run-flat wheels with no tubes. Its total weight was twenty-three kilograms. When it was folded down, Sue could pick up one end by its handle and pull it along on its wheels. And I found it at just the right time too. The blue electric wheelchair I'd been using had served me well, but, by then, it had seen better days and many of its parts were worn out.

My new scooter was yellow. I picked that colour because it was bright and I like yellow for a vehicle. The first brand-new car I bought was a bright yellow Mazda RX7. I loved driving that little sports car. Zoom-zoom! I now had a new yellow vehicle.

***

After I booked the flights, I explained to the travel agent that I needed wheelchair assistance and that I'd be taking my electric mobility scooter as luggage. She was very helpful and efficient in dealing with my requests. I had to answer the airline's questions about my needs and give them the details of my mobility device. I was able to answer easily as I'd learned quite a bit about flying with mobility aids by then.

My old collapsible blue wheelchair weighed thirty kilograms. It used a very heavy dry cell gel battery to power it. The two lighter collapsible parts of the wheelchair were very carefully tied together with the battery for air transport. Two of the wheels on one of the parts had inflatable tyres. I travelled with spare tubes, wheels and a pump. When I first took it overseas to Egypt and Jordan, Dennis was there to help us carry and lift it. My new yellow scooter seemed to be easier and better.

For the Norway trip, I gave the details of the yellow scooter to the travel agent so that she could pass the information on to Thai Airways. I said that my mobility device when collapsed down measured a hundred centimetres long, forty-five centimetres wide and forty-five centimetres high. I gave her the weight of the scooter and said it had a dry cell lithium battery. I also said that I had a material safety data sheet (MSDS) for it and photos. The photos showed the scooter upright, collapsed down and what it was like when someone was moving it. (Photos 2.1.5, 2.1.6 and 2.1.7)

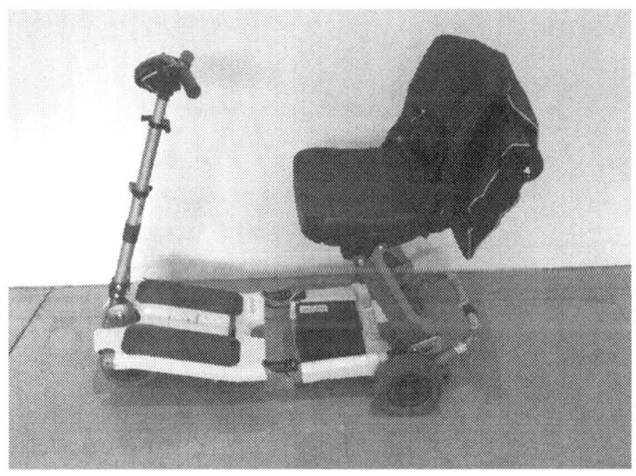

Photo 2.1.5 My Luggie scooter (upright)

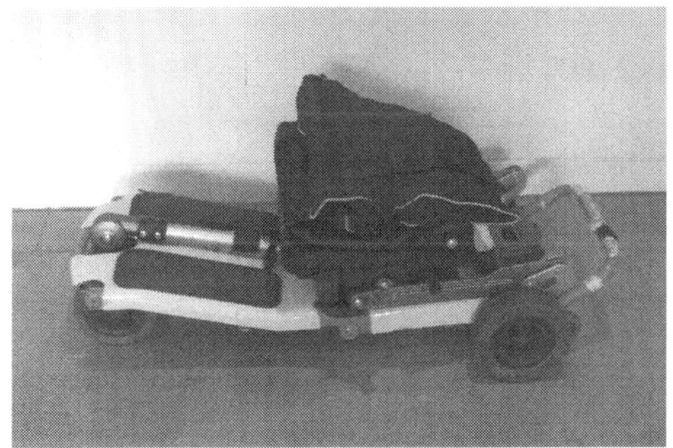

Photo 2.1.6 My Luggie scooter (collapsed)

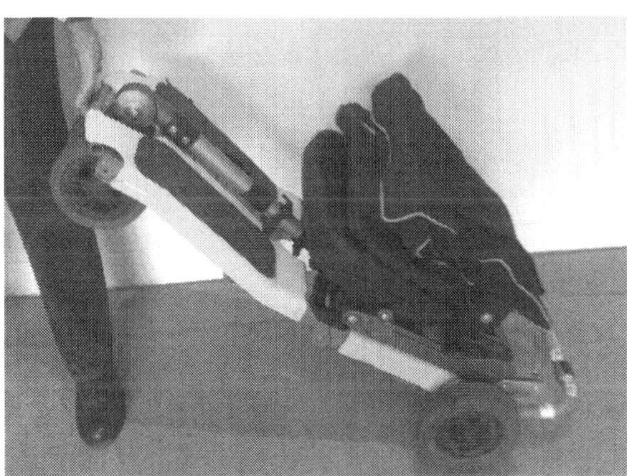

Photo 2.1.7 My Luggie scooter (being moved)

Then I answered the questions in the travel agent's email about my wheelchair assistance needs. The questions and my answers were:

Q. Can you walk up or down airline steps?
A. No

Q. Do you need assistance to get to your seat in the aircraft?
A. No

Q. Do you need help with meals and toileting while aboard?
A. No

Q. Do you have someone travelling with you to help?
A. Yes

By 16 February, I'd paid for our air tickets with credit cards and the travel agent had sent us our e-ticket, itinerary and receipt. We were booked and confirmed to leave on Thursday, 1 September and return on Sunday, 25 September. We would be away for a total of twenty-five days.

I usually liked to travel for less than thirty days at a time and the four-week time constraint for my infusions worked well with that. I was very happy to have finally made a booking. But I wasn't able to do any other work on the trip for a little while. My mind was occupied with something else.

Earlier in January, in the middle of thinking about flights, I'd had a skin lesion removed. It was very small, about three millimetres wide, on my left little toe. It was a funny spot for a spot, I thought, and it looked a bit odd.

I saw a dermatologist and he excised it on 13 January. He rang me six days later to tell me the results. We were driving to Geelong when he called. Mum was in the back of the car because she'd come down for the Australian Open tennis championships and my birthday. We had the old blue wheelchair in the boot. We were taking it to a repair place near Geelong to get it fixed to use as a backup. I remember it all so clearly. My dermatologist asked, 'Is this a good time to talk?'

After a little hesitation, I answered, 'Yes, thanks.'

'Maureen, the pathology report says that it was a Level 1 melanoma… You need to have it excised more widely. Which plastic surgeon would you like to see?' I knew that he meant it was a malignant skin cancer and that it needed wider excision as soon as possible. I asked whom he'd recommend. He suggested a surgeon associated with the melanoma unit, and his secretary made an appointment for me.

The sins of my youth were coming back to bite me. My days of sunbaking, bikini-wearing and surfboard-riding had already shown their effects on my skin; I'd already had several non-malignant skin cancers removed. It's a common story for many Australians.

But what an odd spot, I thought again. On my little toe. How much sun had it seen in its life? Apparently, it wasn't so unusual after all. I was the second person that week to present with it!

The area was more widely excised by my plastic surgeon on 17 February, five weeks after the original excision. That was well within the ideal recommended time of six weeks. The melanoma was small, early and had a very low level of malignancy. It had probably been a complete cure with the first excision. All I needed after the wider excision was a regular follow-up.

I must admit, I was very anxious about having the wider excision done as soon as possible. The appointment on 17 February was the earliest one I could get with that plastic surgeon, and I thought he'd just look at it and then book me in for the surgery on another, later date. But, instead, he excised the area on the same day. I was also worried about getting up and back down the twenty steps to his rooms. But there was no need to worry about that either. His secretary let me in through the car park of the building, where there was a lift. I was able to ride my scooter up to his rooms.

After that, I was back on the job for the trip bookings again. There was much more to do.

I took out travel insurance to cover the September travel period. I'd been relying on credit cards to cover the flight tickets for the few weeks in the meantime, and then the melanoma turned up. My travel insurance policy with my private health insurer, HCF, covered me for emergencies but not those related to multiple sclerosis or melanoma. I was happy enough with that. I thought real emergencies due to those two things would be most unlikely. I also insured my scooter for loss or damages.

I didn't book anything else with travel agents after the flights. I went back to my laptop and the internet, with maps and books spread out across my desk.

The flight was booked. The cruise package was booked, with its one night in a hotel. That left just ten days out of the twenty-five to work out. However, working out those ten days wouldn't be as quick as I'd thought it would be. I wanted to check everything properly and also do the 'Norway in a Nutshell' side trip.

CHAPTER 2

PLANNING AND BOOKING

The 'Norway in a Nutshell' trip – I'd seen that written about so many times as I was planning our holiday. 'The Nutshell' or 'something in a Nutshell' was everywhere. I was hooked straight away. It might have been the idea of capturing so much natural beauty in one neat parcel, the efficiency of it all, or the possibility of being bathed in stunning scenery, or both of those things, that initially allured me. But I was hooked.

Each time I looked at what was involved in doing the Nutshell, there was a problem. There wasn't just one form of transport to go on, there were many. That certainly made it more interesting, but also more worrying for me. There were many unknowns and a lot of coordination to link the flow of transport together. I couldn't work it out quickly. It was a challenge, and I relished challenges and solving problems. I really wanted to go on the Nutshell and I was determined to find a way.

I did worry that my mobility problems would cause difficulties accessing all the forms of transport involved. There were also a lot of changeovers from one kind of transport to another.

To confuse things even more, there were many variations of the Nutshell. Some of the trips went for two days and others for five. There were different routes and different stops. I couldn't just gloss over it any more. I had to get right into the detail to understand exactly what was involved and to work out how we'd do it.

My *Lonely Planet Norway* guidebook helped me start to narrow things down. It said:

> Although most visitors do 'Norway in a Nutshell' from either Oslo or Bergen, you can do a mini version. This circular route from Flåm – boat to Gudvangen, bus to Voss, train to Myrdal, then train down the spectacular Flåmsbana railway to Flåm – is truly the kernel within the nutshell and takes in all the most dramatic elements.*

That was it – 'the kernel'. It was an opportunity to see the best Norway had to offer in a short time – and we didn't have that much time outside the cruise. The kernel, the best of the best, brilliant!

All I needed then was a map to help with my planning and booking. I couldn't find a map of the Nutshell, let alone one of the kernel. So I made one of my own. I used that map to refer back to and show Sue. (Photo 2.2.1)

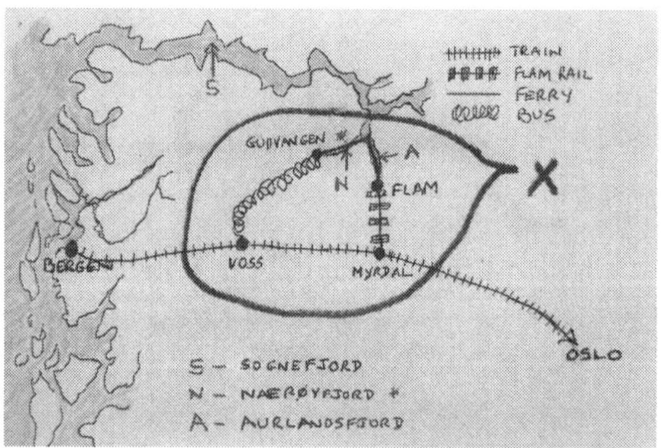

Photo 2.2.1 Map of the kernel in the Nutshell route

That makes it much easier, I thought. I could see the most important part of the Nutshell route, the part that I had to try to fit in. I knew what was an absolute 'must'.

Sue was a bit bewildered by my explanations of what I'd done with my day when she came home from golf or food shopping. 'What is this 'Norway in a Nutshell' business again that you're trying to work out?' I thought I'd explained it. This time, I got the new rough map out and showed her the kernel route that I'd just discovered.

*Reproduced with permission from Norway, 4th edn., Lonely Planet © 2008, Lonely Planet

'You can see it here really easily,' I said. 'There's a train journey, a bus trip and a ferry trip. And you can go in either direction.'

Sue's eyes glazed over a little as she said, 'Oh, okay.' She knew I'd work it out.

I spent time on the Nutshell trip just about every day. Each segment of the Nutshell involved a different form of transport, each with its own timetable. However, to make good progress along the route without hours of delay and waiting, the times had to fit with each other.

I also needed to resolve when, how long and from which direction we'd go on the Nutshell, including the kernel. I had to know that before I could do any other bookings.

Would we do the trip from Oslo or from Bergen? I found out that the Myrdal and Voss train stations were on the main line between Bergen and Oslo. That was wonderful. I'd planned that we'd return from Bergen to Oslo by train anyway. That train trip itself was supposed to include beautiful scenery.

Google Earth helped me see the kernel terrain. It was very mountainous and there were fjords there. It terms of planning, knowing that wasn't much help really and probably made it worse.

The Nutshell area was much closer to Bergen. It was only an hour or two away. It seemed logical to go there from Bergen. That would be at the end of the trip. I thought, yes, we'd stay in Bergen for a few days after finishing the cruise there, and then somehow fit in the Nutshell and continue on our way back to Oslo. We'd then fly back home from Oslo, having done a full circle of Norway. That appealed to me.

In the middle of all of this thinking in February and March, Carolyn rang. 'I've just been talking online, well, writing online, really, live to Norway. I've found a very helpful travel agent in Norway – Helena. She's organising our trip for us. I type what I want, wait a few seconds and she replies in English. She's in Bergen. That's where their office is.'

Carolyn told me that Helena had said, 'Carolyn, we are very pleased to be helping you.'

'And Helena answered all of my questions quickly and easily.'

I asked for Helena's email address. Carolyn sent it to me with the itinerary that Helena had prepared for her and all the other information she'd received. They were going on the Nutshell trip too. I thought I'd cut the time required to do all the bookings and get the Nutshell times coordinated by a local. I'd try dealing with Helena as well.

It started out reasonably well with a detailed itinerary. Then I realised that my itinerary was much the same as Carolyn's. I thought it looked like a *pro forma*, where you just add names. Nevertheless, I continued with Helena.

On the itinerary, Helena suggested a hotel in Oslo and one in Bergen, some day tours, two airport transfers and a Nutshell trip, all without specific dates.

I said we didn't want hotel rooms but that we wanted to stay in self-catering apartments or apartment hotels. Helena replied that they didn't book apartments, only hotel rooms. Oh, okay, I thought, I'll do that part myself.

It was funny that I tried a travel agent to help with those bookings. I'd sometimes used travel agents before and sometimes I'd just booked everything myself. I thought it was probably because our trip to Egypt and Jordan was booked as a package from Australia through a travel agent. It was a small group tour and the agent did everything. It was wonderful and very successful. It was so easy to just check the itinerary, pay the bill and go. That travel agent only dealt in small group tours to four countries. Norway wasn't one of them.

Our trip to Antarctica was also all organised by a travel agent. It was an all-inclusive package with a cruise including arrangements from Australia. We didn't want to add anything else on. So that was easy too.

The trip bookings before that, in 2007, to London, Portugal, France and Honolulu, I'd done all that myself. I'd even used Frequent Flyer points to do most of the airline bookings. I did all the other bookings online for six of us. There was the canal-boat hire, the car hire, the hotels and apartments. So, I was capable of doing it. I'd just got out of the habit. Yes, I was lulled into what I thought was the easy way.

Then I thought again and realised that my reason for doing the bookings to Egypt and Jordan through a travel agent and going on a small group tour, was that it was all very foreign. I forgave myself for taking the easy option then.

However, this trip was to a European country; it wouldn't be foreign. The culture would be similar to ours and speaking English would be okay. I'd done it before. So then I thought, yes, I'll book the accommodation in Norway myself and leave what I thought were the harder things, like transfers, the train and the Nutshell, to Helena.

In my next few emails to Helena, I explained (or thought I did) my mobility needs so she could do more bookings. I didn't think they were complicated. However, that was only the start of me trying to explain what I needed.

When I told people that I used a mobility scooter, they sometimes thought it was like a child's scooter, that you placed one leg on it and pushed with the other. I had to say it was a 'wheel-chair-scooter' for them to understand. However, it was often quite difficult for people to really get it until they saw me on it. I tried to send a photo to Helena but that didn't seem to help. It may not have even reached her.

There were many emails back and forth trying to clarify the situation and my request. I wanted to go on all the forms of transport and take my collapsible scooter with me.

For the Nutshell, Helena said I could *not* go on the ferry boat between Flåm and Gudvangen with a wheelchair-scooter. She also said I could *not* go on the bus between Gudvangen and Voss. However, I could go on the Flåm Line. But, at Flåm, I'd need to either arrive or leave on a larger ferry that took wheelchairs and that went on the route between Bergen and Flåm as an express commuter ferry. Helena said that trip was called the 'Sognefjord in a Nutshell' trip, another Nutshell.

The information I read in the *Lonely Planet Norway* said the bus went on the Stalheimskleiva road through mountains – the old mail road. The road 'twists and turns down 13 steep and spectacular hairpin bends offering wonderful views' of the gorge and waterfalls. The view from the town at the top, in particular from the hotel at Stalheim, was supposed to be famous too, with the 'best view in Norway'. That bus trip sounded fantastic. But Helena said *no*!

I inquired a bit more about the bus sector. The road was open until near the end of September but from October it closed for winter. We were going at the end of September, but the weather wasn't the reason I was told I couldn't go.

Whenever I tried to find out information about these buses from other sources – whether they'd be able to take my wheelchair-scooter – my inquiries were met with firm replies. 'No, it is an old bus' and 'No, you cannot leave the wheelchair-scooter or luggage at Voss and come back for it later.'

So it was a total *no* to that one bus trip between the Gudvangen ferry stop and Voss Station.

At least the other trip that Helena suggested covered the Flåm Line. Now there was the ferry trip to resolve. From my maps, I could see that the ferry from Flåm, on the route that Helena was proposing, went through the Sognefjord to Bergen. Sognefjord was the longest and deepest fjord in Norway. Perhaps that was the answer then. I almost booked it but it still didn't seem right. To do that ferry trip would mean we'd be going on a circular route back to Bergen again where we started.

'But that leaves out the UNESCO World Heritage Nærøyfjørd,' I emailed back to Helena. 'It wouldn't be World Heritage listed if it wasn't something we had to see.' There was no change in her recommendation. I found it very frustrating.

I emailed Mariana at the local tourist office in Flåm next. Her written English was a little difficult but she was very helpful. Mariana said yes, I could go on the ferry from Flåm to Gudvangen with my wheelchair-scooter, but I couldn't go upstairs on the boat.

I'd have to stay downstairs. At Gudvangen, I could *not* get the bus to Voss. (That last part was consistent with what Helena had said.) The bus didn't take wheelchairs. I'd have to return to Flåm on the same ferry. Mariana then told me the times of the ferries. She said that I'd have to catch the 1.10 p.m. ferry from Flåm and the 4 p.m. ferry back – that was the last one of the day. The ferry trip each way took two hours and ten minutes, almost four-and-a-half hours in all. It also meant that it would be late when we got back to Flåm.

Thinking it through again, I could see that on the day we wanted to go to Nærøyfjørd, we had to arrive in Flåm before 1 p.m. and then stay the night when we got back. Carolyn and her friends were staying the night in Flåm. That way of doing the Nutshell was starting to seem possible.

I explained to Helena what the local tourist office had told me. I asked her to make a booking for me that included a return ferry component and the Flåm Line part of their 'Norway in a Nutshell' tour. She said she'd have to talk to her supervisor and then get back to me.

Later that day, Sue came home from playing golf. I asked her, 'How did you go today?'

'We were coming first until we were pipped. We got thirty-four points.'

'Oh, okay,' I said.

'How has your day been?' Sue asked.

'You won't believe all these emails about trying to do the Nutshell.' I gave Sue a shortened version of where I was up to and what trouble I was having.

'Let's see what she comes back with. What would you like for dinner? I'm about to go out to do the shopping. I'll just go to Coles and Thomas Dux. I'll go to the markets tomorrow. Did you eat all your lunch that I left? Is there anything you want?' Sue did all the food shopping, preparation and cooking. Sometimes I was so carried away with doing trip research at my computer, that I'd forget to have the lunch Sue sometimes left for me. She was usually home around lunchtime to make it for me on most days.

'Yes, I had lunch, thanks. Oh, I've run out of light pink printer ink. Could you get some from Office Works while you're out?'

'I might do that tomorrow. The traffic will be bad. It'll be school pick-up time if I go there after shopping. I have all day tomorrow to do things like that for you. Can you wait?'

'Yes, sure, it's not urgent. Tomorrow will be fine.'

'Okay, bye, will be about an hour.'

Helena emailed back the next day and said that she wasn't allowed to make a booking for me on that ferry as part of the 'Norway in a Nutshell' tour. She said her travel company didn't want to be responsible for the booking in case something went wrong for me on my wheelchair-scooter.

By this time, I only had about two other things to be booked with Helena. I started with about six and as time went on, I kept deleting them. The transfers from airports, the hotels, and the sightseeing trips were all crossed off the list.

With Helena, that was the end. I'd had enough. I thanked her for her help and said I'd manage it all myself now. So, from that point on, I did all the bookings and even the deeper investigation on my own. I wasn't at all convinced that we had to stay on the ferry and do two trips on the same route.

I was completely hooked by the Nutshell and was enthusiastically negotiating the challenge; the fact that I was being told that I could *not* do something put up my red flag and I became even more determined to do it. I had learned that defying 'no' could reap huge rewards. During my first few years of high school, I was told that I could *not* study the highest levels of mathematics or science because girls didn't do that. Girls couldn't do those subjects and didn't need to anyway! Defying that 'no' led to many wonderful rewards.

My research into each part of the Nutshell trip took a long time. I tried getting in touch with disability organisations for help, as well as some websites and contacts, and Googled my queries on the internet. I had been doing this finer part of the planning and booking process for weeks with no success.

My last idea was to look for help in another way. Once a month, I wrote an article for a disability website called *DiVine*, a name arising out from the idea of creating a disability grapevine. The Victorian government's Office for Disability established and managed this site with the help of an editor. I thought I'd write an article about my difficulties getting information about the Nutshell and ask readers if they knew something about it. I wrote a five-hundred-word article in March and submitted it to the editor.

It was titled 'Accessibility in Norway?' I explained the cruise that I'd booked and how I expected accessibility on board the ship for my small electric scooter to be all right. Then, under the sub-heading 'Many Changeovers', I wrote of what I by now thought of as the famous (it certainly was in my mind) Norway in a Nutshell trip. I wrote that I had no real idea about the accessibility of any of the forms of transport and was especially concerned about being able to do the changeovers.

I was so worried about the changeovers because we had to get the scooter, our luggage and me between them. Would I be able to ride the scooter or would I have to walk? How far was it and what was the surface like? If the scooter couldn't get over the ground, how would we all get there? Some *DiVine* readers were wheelchair users and would easily understand, but I went into a bit more detail for the general reader.

In my article, I tried to keep my quest for information broad to start with. I wrote, 'What is it really like to travel in Norway with a disability? I wonder if anyone has some first-hand information, especially around the Nutshell.'

The editor replied quickly. He thought my article didn't fit the general brief for the *DiVine* website. He said it was a bit esoteric, and suggested I write something when I get back about what happened. Feeling deflated by not being able to have the article published, I went back to finding out information on my own again.

Most days I'd go to my desk on my red indoor electric wheelchair, start up the computer, look at websites and send emails. Sometimes I'd stop and do some exercises. My desk held a printer/

scanner to my right beside the laptop in front of me. On my left was a pile of paperwork. My calendar sat on top of it. A fold-back clip held a few pages of notes. Finding out how to do the Nutshell had its own life now, it seemed.

It was becoming more than a challenge. It was sometimes like something was broken and I *had* to fix it! Besides, I couldn't book anything else until I booked that part of the trip.

Sue came home from golf. As she came in the door she said, 'I'm ho-ome,' as she usually did. It was about time I stopped for the day.

'How did you go today?' I asked.

'I couldn't putt to save myself,' Sue said.

'Oh, okay.'

'What have you been up to?

'Just trying to do the Nutshell bookings again.'

'You're like a dog with a bone sometimes, aren't you? Have you been out for a walk or a swim yet today?'

'Yes, I went for a walk this morning. Just along the front and back. It wasn't too hot. I'll try and go for a swim in the next few days, if it's nice.'

'Good.'

A few days after I submitted the rejected article, we went away for about two weeks. It was timely because I really did need a break from working on the trip. It was starting to drive me bananas. Sometimes I get too focused and have to be rescued from myself.

Besides, I wanted to be with my mother for her eighty-second birthday, which was coming up on 11 March. A visit to her place first would kick off the two-week trip away. We drove the roughly one thousand kilometres north to the NSW Central Coast, where I grew up. I was looking forward to catching up with Mum.

Sue drove us up there in her Subaru Forester wagon. That small SUV was reasonably good for transporting the scooter and Sue did all the driving. I'd stopped driving some years ago. After a few breaks along the way, we made it to Mum's in about eleven-and-a-half hours. The Hume Freeway was fabulous, with no traffic lights to obey after we left Melbourne until we reached the Pennant Hills Road Exit, nine hundred kilometres away.

Mum lived in a nice place overlooking a lake; she called her home 'Tranquil Waters'. Dad had left the family many years ago. Mum was a good businesswoman and worked well into her seventies. She had accomplished a great deal. Certainly a lot more than the teacher who successfully discouraged her from finishing high school expected, I'm sure. That was such a shame. She took herself to a Technical and Further Education (TAFE) college much later, when she was in her fifties, and sailed through with distinction. She became a hardworking real estate agent and auctioneer, and was also a local character. Mum had a personality of her very own, a real trick, and I was proud of her.

When we were up at Mum's on the day of her birthday, the television was turned on to ABC News 24 for the noon news. Suddenly, I couldn't believe what I was seeing in front of my eyes. I called out to everyone, 'Oh, no! You have to come and have a look at this! Mum, Sue! It's terrible.'

I'd heard about the large earthquake in Japan on the breakfast news. Then, there on the TV screen, the massive tsunami that followed it was moving in towards land in front of my eyes. I could see towns with cars and houses in the foreground and open fields off to one side. Behind them, in the background, was a massive wave of water rolling in. The huge amount of water was moving fast and heading straight for them. I saw cars trying to get away, rushing one way and then turning another way. Other cars just seemed to be travelling along unaware of what was about to happen to them. I knew there was probably no way that the people inside them would survive. I felt that it was wrong somehow – watching. Watching what was about to happen to these people.

I sent Carolyn an SMS that said, 'Turn on ABC News 24 if u can. A terrible tsunami, happening in Japan, right now.'

The news unfolded in the days that followed. There were twenty thousand people reported killed and damage to the Fukushima nuclear plant had set off a nuclear crisis in the country. I'd never been to Japan. Sue said she was there in the 1970s. I really felt sad for the Japanese people. It would probably be a while before we'd be thinking of going on a trip there.

Mum told me about her trip to Japan, when that country's first world expo was on in 1970. She'd left her tour group in Osaka and went on her own to Hiroshima for the day. She'd caught the bullet train and all the Japanese people around her were very friendly. Many wanted to practice speaking English with her, both children and adults. Some people on the tour had been worried that she wouldn't get back in time to catch the flight home. But she had no problems and loved being able to see the place, as well as all the adventure involved in going there.

I told Mum a little bit about trying to book the Nutshell side trip and that there were a lot of different little steps involved. 'Oh, well, love, remember, inch by inch, everything's a cinch.' She had a key ring in the shape of a small brass ruler with inches marked on it and that saying inscribed on it!

Next, we went up to Queensland. I wanted to check how my house was going and hoped that the weather had cooled down enough for me to be there.

I'd travelled to Queensland quite a bit. When I was working there, I'd bought a house on the Sunshine Coast, north of Brisbane. I love being there, but since I'd developed MS I hadn't been able to go when the weather was hot. I have heat-sensitivity, as do at least seventy-five per cent of other people with MS.

***

I couldn't believe how sensitive my body had become to heat, to hot weather and to high temperatures around me. I used to do a lot of outdoor activities in the sun without any problems. But, with MS, I could immediately tell when the temperature went over 24°C. It was almost as if I was a living thermometer and could feel and sense every degree over that.

When it was hot, it felt as if my body had melted. If I'd missed the warning signs (learned by experience) and let myself get too hot, I'd hardly be able to move. The effort required to even lift my hand became too much. I'd just have to lie down, get some help to cool down or wait for the temperature to change.

I'd tried out a lot of cooling devices. Everything from fans (all varieties), wet neckties, cooling vests, cooling towels, water air coolers, air conditioning, you name it! I was still open to trying something new but, really, the best thing for me was to avoid the heat altogether. Next best was sitting quietly in air conditioning.

To manage the extreme heat, I had to plan and organise any activities that required my body to move. That meant things such as walking and showering, knowing where to sit to keep cool and when to do things.

I imagine the heat melts the myelin lining my nerves (or whatever myelin is left) and they end up not being able to conduct anything and stopped working. I tried to have Christmas up on the Sunshine Coast one year, and it became so hot that I collapsed on the lounge and couldn't move for a while. Mum was staying with me at the time and she said, 'Oh dear, love, does this happen very often?'

To have such a strong reaction to the weather is very strange. Another strange but absolutely fascinating thing is a related subject, the 'geography' of MS.

I love geography. I was quite good at it in school and still enjoy learning about it. That's probably where my love of maps comes from. So I was really fascinated when I saw a map of the world showing bands of latitudes in different colours that corresponded to rates of MS around the world. The number of people with MS increased the further away they were from the equator, both north and south. Some studies spoke of a 40° latitude divide, others quoted 45° to 65° lines of latitude as the band with the highest prevalence of MS. The prevalence in that band was 60 to 100 per 100,000 people. Prevalence was directly proportional to the distance from the equator. Fascinating!

The disease is virtually unknown near the equator and is highest in northern Europe, the UK, southern Scandinavia, northern USA and southern Canada. It's also highest at similar latitudes in the south – in southern Australia and New Zealand.

There's an east/west divide too. MS is rare in Asian countries such as Japan and China, and all the prevalence bands are in the west. Another study revealed that MS is also virtually unknown among Inuit and other indigenous peoples. It really was a Celtic or 'Viking disease', as it has been called in the past.

These findings have led researchers to suggest that there are genetic and environmental factors involved. The environmental factors could be infections, the amount of sunlight or daylight available, diet and perhaps soil. And it's significant where a person grows up; this is what determines risk, not where they might have moved to later. Latitude is more strongly related to MS than any other risk factor.

In Australia, on the eastern side, the highest rate is in Tasmania, the lowest in Queensland (very low) and NSW, where I grew up, is between the two.

I usually go to the Sunshine Coast when it isn't hot, in the winter months of June, July and August. The maximum temperature at that time is in the low twenties. It's also very cold in Melbourne at that time, and I join the regular 'invasion from the south'. Some warmth is nice.

***

We drove from Mum's to Newcastle Airport to catch a flight to Brisbane. We flew with Jetstar. This would be a good test of travelling with my new mobility scooter. Even though I'd flown with Jetstar before, the scooter arrangements were different at each airport and I learned something new every time.

At Brisbane Airport, I hired a suitable rental car so that Sue (and I) could lift the scooter up into the boot without too much trouble. The scooter also had to fit into the space easily and preferably go straight in to avoid lifting it later. The lower the loading lip, the better it was – that way, there was more rolling and less lifting. All on board, we drove the approximately 120 kilometres north from Brisbane to the Sunshine Coast.

Up in south-eastern Queensland, in March, I hoped the cool coastal breezes along the Sunshine Coast would kick in and keep temperatures in the low twenties. At that time of year, it was, very oddly, too hot in Melbourne, where temperatures could reach into the forties, with bushfires in the news.

The house on the Sunshine Coast was fine and I just relaxed.

Well, that's not entirely true. John, who lived up there and had been a friend for many years, was not well when we arrived. He was partially blind, fiercely independent and lived on his own. Despite his poor sight, he still travelled a lot. We took him to see his specialist to have some pathology tests, but he became so unwell that Sue had to drive him to hospital while we were up there.

John really loved to travel. He told many wonderful stories. I recalled that he'd said he'd been to Norway as a young man, working on merchant ships. I also recalled him saying that he wasn't sure how he got from Bergen in Norway to Sweden but the Flåm Line was clear in his mind. 'Oh, that train journey, the Flåm, was just marvellous.' I can still hear John's words. He spoke beautifully.

After thinking more about what John had said, I was even more determined to visit at least the Flåm part of the Nutshell. I couldn't stop thinking about it. I couldn't switch my mind off the unbooked parts of the trip. So I started to look at all the bookings again while we were away on the Sunshine Coast.

This time, I thought I'd start with the low-lying fruit and do some easy bookings. I needed to feel as if I was making some progress in all of this. I wanted to book something!

I had to book the nights in Oslo before the flight north to Longyearbyen, the nights in Bergen after disembarking from the ship and then the days finding our way back to Oslo to fly home. In among the last leg of travel, we'd do the Nutshell. I'd allow two days for it. I thought I'd just forget how we were going to do it for the moment. I'd leave that for later.

In Oslo, at the beginning of the trip, we wanted a self-catering apartment or hotel. We were going to be there for five nights and wanted to feel like we were living in Oslo for a short while. We wanted to shop at the local supermarket, visit food markets, go to the local liquor store and choose our own food. We wanted the space of an apartment, with some privacy and control over our meals. We wanted to experience the feel of the place, including its fresh food.

I just Googled 'apartments in Oslo' and soon found the Frogner House Apartments. I contacted them by email and asked about accessibility. Were there any steps? Was there lift access if there were stairs? Was there a walk-in shower, not one over a bathtub?

Fredrik at Frogner House replied, 'We welcome you to stay with us. There are only three stairs. There is no bath only a shower.'

I emailed back straight away and asked him, 'Do you mean three steps or three staircases with each of the stairs having about twelve steps to them, meaning thirty-six steps all together?'

'Thank you for your quick reply,' Fredrik emailed back. 'There are not thirty-six, just three small steps at the entry.'

The place seemed good. The shower was a walk-in one and there was a lift in the building. The one-bedroom apartment was in central Oslo, near a park and the Royal Palace. It was close to public transport, a supermarket and shops.

On 14 March, I booked the Frogner House Apartment at Arbinsgate 3 for five nights from 2–7 September. At last, I'd made some more progress.

Then I started thinking about the transfers. How to get from the airport to the apartment in Oslo? My mind always jumps to what I think is the easiest way. That is, just get a taxi. In my reading – the *Lonely Planet Norway* guide – that option wasn't even mentioned. Gardermoen International Airport was fifty kilometres north of Oslo. The high-speed train (Flytoget) and the shuttle bus service (Flybussen) were both explained in the guide. But what about wheelchair access? I left that one for the time being.

We flew back to Newcastle, drove to Mum's and soon after drove back to Melbourne.

Once home again, wanting to have something else concrete to show for all my time spent planning the trip, I decided to book the hotel for the end of the trip, once again in Oslo. I found a hotel adjacent to the fast-train link to the airport. I hoped we'd have worked out the transport system by that stage. The hotel was on the other side of the city to the Frogner Apartments, so that would be different. It overlooked a new opera house and a fjord. It seemed an ideal location.

I used a hotel-booking website and saw one of their cheap advanced booking deals. It was a four- to five-star hotel and, according to the information supplied on the website, it passed all my accessibility requirements. On 25 March, I booked the Thon Hotel Opera in Oslo for one night, 23 September. So now the last night of the trip was booked.

That day was also momentous because it was the starting date for Sue's golf competition. Sue had been practising at the driving range more often than usual in readiness for it. The driving range was only a short way away. The competition would last until the end of May. She'd be playing golf more often and I had more time to do investigations and bookings for the trip.

Booking the accommodation in Bergen was next. From my reading, I knew there were a lot of hills and mountains in the city. I wanted a place on flat ground, near the harbour and close to the centre of town.

I started by looking at where I thought the ship would berth. I looked at the maps in the *Lonely Planet Norway* guide. I saw a Hurtigruten symbol at a one of the docks to the south of the city. It seemed to be about five kilometres away from the town centre. If that were correct, there would be another transfer to organise. That shouldn't be difficult, I thought, as a whole shipload of passengers would be disembarking. It was something I could organise while on the ship or we could just get a taxi.

All the apartments advertised for rent on the internet were either long-stay or on the side of hills with cobbled streets. None of them jumped out at me. I thought, Oh well, we'd only be there for a few days. Bergen is smaller than Oslo. Perhaps a hotel will do after all.

I read a few travel brochures, the *Lonely Planet Norway* and had a look on the internet. I liked the sound and look of the Augustin Hotel near the docks in Bergen. I earmarked that in my mind, though I still wasn't sure.

On 28 March, we received the sad news that John had died that day in hospital. We were upset, but when we spoke to his family and friends they said they were pleased that he was able to stay in his own home for so long. They told us he'd been deteriorating for some time. He'd lived well into his eighties and had enjoyed every year of it. It was better for him to go that way. His funeral would be in few days' time and we were going.

Meantime, back at my desk, the emails were coming in from tourist offices and tour operators. I was making enquiries about the Nutshell again. 'You cannot go on the tour with a wheelchair,' they said again.

At one stage, our communication in English seemed to be at odds. 'You can use our wheelchair on the Flåm Line but you cannot take it away with you when you get off.'

I explained that I didn't want to use their wheelchair on the Flåm Line and take it away with me. I had my own wheelchair-scooter. I just wanted to carry it on the train along with our luggage.

That was the other issue to consider. What about the luggage? If we were going to be changing forms of transport we'd have to carry our luggage as well, especially if we were on our way to Oslo and home. The information about the Nutshell that I was reading warned of difficulties taking luggage on the trip. It said storage was limited along the way.

At one stage, after considering this problem, I wondered about a day trip from Bergen. Leave the baggage in the room at the hotel, stay another night. Travel with just the scooter. We'd have only one medium suitcase anyway. We always share one bag to save on items for Sue to manage. When I investigated this idea, it seemed it was possible but it would be a very long day, involving at least twelve hours of travel. It didn't seem sensible to go twice on the same route either.

I found the Norwegian State Railways (NSB) timetable and booking service. I could see the trains from Bergen to Voss, Myrdal, Flåm and Oslo. But I could only see the times for the next three months. Anything after three months was blank. I had to wait until after the third week of June to be able to see the actual times for the third week of September. There seemed to be plenty of choices each day though.

When Sue came home at the end of her golfing day, I, as usual, asked how she went. 'It was very windy, a three-club wind.' Then, 'How are you getting on with the trip?' When I tried to explain my frustration, we had to sit down and go through the highlighted map again. For a simple side-trip, it seemed to be getting very complicated. I didn't take Sue through all the details. That would have been too much. Then I remembered two other things that I'd done that day.

'Oh, I was able to change those tickets to the MSO (Melbourne Symphony Orchestra) and for that play, because we'll be away when they're on. I rang and we'll be able to exchange the MTC (Melbourne Theatre Company) tickets at the box office on the night but the MSO tickets have to be posted off. They're on the shelf near the front door, ready to be posted.'

'Great, that's good.' Sue listened to my daily report and then she got on with things. 'I'm going to do a load of washing. Is there anything you can think of that needs washing?'

'No, just what's in the basket, thanks.'

Also sometime in March, in the middle of my bookings and Nutshell obsession, I received a letter in the mail from my neurologist. When I'd seen him in early December the previous year, he'd spoken to me about a special blood test that was about to become available for MS patients who were receiving Tysabri. The test was still going through its approval process at the time. He wrote:

> The blood test is to look for JC virus antibodies, as about 50% of the population have antibodies, and the others do not.
>
> Patients who have the antibodies are a 1:1,000 risk of PML

(Progressive Multifocal Leukoencephalopathy). If you do not have positive antibodies, the risk of PML is negligible.

PML is a life-threatening condition. Most people who develop it die. The test was part of a research project at Royal Melbourne Hospital. The full title of the project was 'Epidemiology of Anti-JCV Antibody Prevalence in Multiple Sclerosis Patients: JEMS Study'.

On 30 March, I had my blood test for JC virus antibodies at the hospital, just before my four-weekly intravenous infusion of Tysabri. The nurse sent the blood to the US, via Singapore she said, for testing. It could be six weeks before I knew the result. Well, I thought, that will be useful to know before I travel overseas!

***

I knew about the JC virus. My neurologist had told me about the risks before I started Tysabri two years before. The risks were that I could have an anaphylactic reaction and I could develop PML.

That first Tysabri infusion flashed through my mind. It was in February 2009 and I was very anxious on that first visit to the chemo day centre. I was terrified that I might have some immediate reaction to the new drug right then and there on day one. If that didn't happen, I was terrified that I might actually get PML in the time that followed. That would be terrible. I could go into a vegetative state and die. My usually normal blood pressure was high, at 170 on 110, when it was measured before starting the infusion. I think the nurse, Jen, who took my blood pressure knew I was anxious and she just chatted on as she was doing her checks.

What could I do now, anyway, here in the Day Surgery/Chemotherapy Unit? I'd thought about it all very seriously before I said yes to my neurologist and before I went to the unit. I'd checked that there was a good medical emergency team on call at all times. I knew there was an Intensive Care Unit within the complex of private and public hospitals of the Royal Melbourne Hospital campus. The potential benefit was worth the risk, I thought.

Although I felt entitled to feel anxious, I also knew that anxiety was a symptom of MS. The whole idea of the infusion made it worse! I just had to sit there and think of something else – perhaps try to read the book that I'd brought with me.

Nothing adverse happened at the first infusion and nothing has happened since. My blood pressure returned to normal and I left after two-and-a-half uneventful hours.

There was no test for the JC virus two years ago. It was just a risk. A fairly significant risk, though. And now there was this chance to test how bad the risk was. If it was positive, the risk was as high as one in one thousand. If it was negative, the risk was close to zero. I had a fifty per cent chance of having the virus anyway as part of the normal population. It would certainly be good to know the result, what my real chances were, before I went overseas.

***

That night, we flew back up to Brisbane to go to John's funeral at Coolum. His family had arranged that a few people would place special objects belonging to John on his coffin during the mass. Sue placed his favourite dark sunglasses, the ones he wore walking and travelling, on to his coffin. 'The Flåm – marvellous,' I could hear him say.

My yellow scooter travelled on the flights without problems and we were back in Melbourne later the next day. I pressed on with my Nutshell investigations.

The next easiest thing to book, I thought, was the accommodation in Flåm. I asked the local tourist office about that. I asked about places close to the train station and the ferry terminal. I wanted to know how close together they were as well.

In an email from the local tourist office, Mariana told me that the Flåmsbrygga Hotel was 'right next to both the rail terminal and the ferry, within 100 metres.' Using Google Earth I could see the hotel right on the water and the station exactly as described. Mariana went on to say that the Flåmsbrygga Hotel had 'rooms at ground level, so you will not have to go upstairs.' One night there seemed like it could fit in perfectly.

I thought we might arrive in Flåm in time to take our bags to the hotel, quickly book in and be able to catch the 1.10 p.m. ferry. We could then return on the 4 p.m. ferry and be back at the hotel by about 6 p.m. That could all happen if we followed through with the idea of taking two trips on the ferry.

What about Bergen? How long to stay there? I'd made an estimate of staying three nights. I thought that we'd leave by train on the fourth day after arriving from our cruise. The plan was to get to the hotel in Flåm and stay the night. Then get back on the train to Oslo the next day.

I still wasn't absolutely sure exactly how we'd end up going on the Nærøyfjord. The plan at that stage was to do two trips on the Flåm Line, one down, one up. It seemed we couldn't get back to the main train line any other way. I had accepted that the bus to Voss was a definite no. But I wasn't going to take any more no's!

I'd already thought about how I might access the ferry. I thought I'd ride the scooter from Flåm Station to the hotel, with Sue walking; We'd book in and leave our suitcase there. Then I'd ride the scooter to the ferry stop, again with Sue walking. Once there, I'd get off the scooter, stand at the ferry stop with my walking stick and wait. I thought both Sue and I would keep an eye out for a chair for me to sit on or something to lean on while I waited. I wasn't allowed to take the scooter on board so Sue could ride the scooter back to the hotel and ask them to mind it. After that, she'd walk back to me at the ferry stop. When the ferry came in, Sue could help me get on and I'd sit on a seat for the trip into the fjord and back.

I thought I'd done enough investigating to make the one-night booking in Flåm and the three-night booking in Bergen. I emailed both hotels, told them about my mobility needs, asked them about the showers and whether there were any stairs, and checked about lifts in the Augustin Hotel in Bergen.

Staff at the hotel in Bergen replied that they had rooms with bathrooms for people with disabilities and they had lifts in the building with no steps or stairs to the room. Perfect. They told me that all I needed to do when I booked online was request the disabled bathroom in the booking request box. However, they also asked me for the measurements of my scooter, saying in one email, 'Our elevators are small ones. We will have to measure them to see if you will fit in.'

I thanked them and sent back the measurements of the scooter. They soon replied. 'We have two elevators. It will not fit in the main one. The second elevator is around the corner and it will fit in there.'

I replied, 'Thank you. Could you please explain where around the corner is? Is the lift in another building?'

They emailed back to say, 'No, the larger elevator is not in another building. It is in a corner around from the front desk.'

I thanked them again and asked one more question. 'Is that the lift that will take me up to the same level where the room with the disabled bathroom is?'

'Yes, of course.'

'Great, thank you, I will book that room online very soon.'

Meantime, the hotel in Flåm had answered my email queries as well. I asked for a room on the ground floor. That's what the local tourist office had recommended because of my mobility problems. I looked at the photos of the hotel on their website. It looked like a two-storey wooden A-framed building, not terribly large, located right on the fjord waterfront. The Flåmsbrygga Hotel said they had a room available on the ground floor, that it was all level, and the shower was a walk-in one, with no bathtub. They also said Flåm Station was about a hundred metres away. Good, I thought. I'll book that soon too.

While investigating accommodation in Norway, and at about the same time, I also found that there was up to twenty per cent discount on hotel accommodation if you purchased a 'Fjord Pass', for about AUD$20. After calculating whether it would be worth it, comparing the new total with the actual already discounted prices for the two hotels, I purchased the pass.

On 8 April, I booked three nights at the Augustin Hotel in Bergen from 19–21 September and one night in Flåm at the Flåmsbrygga Hotel for 22 September. I had to pay the discounted price when we arrived at the hotels and show the pass; both would be at the special price. The names of those last two hotels could go into the travel table that I was putting together. I always put together a table with dates, days, transport, location, accommodation and booking references all recorded. All the accommodation boxes could now be filled in.

What remained to book was the transport from Bergen to Flåm, the kernel part of the Nutshell and then the train to Oslo. That was still the most difficult part to figure out. By that time in the booking process, I needed a rest from it all again. When I start on something, I usually like to finish it. But I had to stop for a while. I do drive myself hard to make sure I do things properly.

I was worried about not being able to manage a situation while we were away. There would be only Sue to help me. I wanted to try and have it all worked out before we left.

Also, by then, Sue had just about had enough of loading the Luggie scooter into the high boot space of the Subaru. Renting other cars made us realise that the height of the boot space was very important for scooter-loading. It was time to talk in detail about what we were going to do about it. I wanted it to be easy for her. We measured the height of the Subaru boot lip. We looked at every car that went past when we were driving. We measured the space and heights in parked cars. We read brochures and visited car showrooms.

We talked about safety too. The Subaru had only one airbag and that was for the driver's seat. There were no ABS brakes.

Keen to get my mind doing things other than thinking about the trip, I made a spreadsheet with all the cars we thought were possibilities. Across the top of the spreadsheet I listed the criteria that we wanted, our wish list: boot space of at least one thousand millimetres in length and width, a low loading lip up to the boot area, driver and passenger seats with easy access, no step up and adjustable height seats, the latest safety features, comfort and suitability for long trips, automatic transmission, diesel fuel, not too big or too long, and snazzy looks. A second-hand or demonstration model with low kilometres would be considered.

I listed various vehicle brands down the left side of the sheet, did some research online and then headed out to test our selections.

We decided that it was a wagon we were after rather than a sedan. There were lots on offer. The wagons that we finally tested were a Volkswagen Golf Wagon, a Skoda Superb and a Subaru Outback.

We went with tape measure, walker and my yellow travel scooter to test them all. Sue did the test-driving.

Our choice in the end was the Volkswagen. There was a demonstration model available that also had dual air-conditioning controls. I thought this would come in very handy for someone with MS and heat intolerance. This feature helped clinch the deal. All we had to do was organise some tinting to reduce the sun's rays and we were away.

The new car was silver and the yellow Luggie scooter fitted in perfectly, rolling in easily with minimal lifting. On my passenger side, I could raise and lower the seat and move it backwards and forwards easily. I also had my own temperature control. The car brakes worked well and there was an airbag in front of me. Sue enjoyed driving this car, and found that loading the scooter was much easier. It was a very good choice, we thought, perfect for our needs.

I was pleased that I didn't have to organise a hire car while we were away in Norway. I'd organised one before for travelling with my blue electric wheelchair. That was on a trip driving around Portugal in 2007, with six of us in all. There were lots of people to help Sue load and unload my mobility equipment then and the criteria were not as strict.

Carolyn left Australia a few days after we bought the new car.

Although she and her friends were going to Norway in June, she left Australia on 22 April. She was going to Germany first and then off on a holiday to Croatia before going to Norway. The Nutshell tour was included in the Norway trip that Helena had organised for all of them. They were fit and able and could manage all the forms of transport. Carolyn offered to take a lot of photos for me, especially of the Nutshell parts. She took a list of questions that I still had and was going to help me figure it all out. My questions were about distances and the kind of terrain that I might encounter. I'd wait until she returned before booking the train from Bergen to Oslo and the other transport parts of the Nutshell.

I also gave Carolyn the names of the hotels I'd just booked in Flåm and Bergen. She said she'd check those out for us too. Carolyn would report back to me in July.

Just a few days after Carolyn had left, Sue and I were in the car park of our apartment block when we ran into our neighbours Ron and Sandra. We said hello and before long we were talking travel. They said they were going on a cruise to Greenland and Iceland, and then over to the coast of Norway to see a few fjords. I asked if they were going on the Flåm Line. Yes, they were. 'The cruise ship anchors at Flåm,' said Ron. 'It goes up the fjord to get there and we've booked an excursion from Flåm.'

I explained that I was trying to find out information about the Nutshell.

'Yes, that's what they called the trip from Flåm,' said Sandra. 'Something about a nutshell.'

Ron said, 'I'll give you the excursion notes. They have something about people with mobility problems doing excursions. There might be something there for you.'

'Thanks,' I said. 'That would be just great.'

I asked them too, when they went, if they could take particular note of the train changeover at Myrdal.

I had trouble thinking through the changeover because I knew the Flåm train was very old. I didn't think that an old train could run on a new line such as the national railway system. The Flåm

Line had its own design and I thought it would have its own station too, like some of the old steam train lines in Australia, such as the Mary Rattler at Gympie. I thought what might happen was that we'd arrive at Myrdal on the regional train from Bergen and then we'd have to find our way to another station, kilometres away. I wanted to know how far it was between the two points.

Sandra said, 'Just Google it.' Yes, thanks, I thought, but I'd already been doing that.

I just said, 'Oh, okay, I'll try that.'

Ron and Sandra were leaving in a few weeks. We still had just over three months to go. They said they'd take note of the trains at Myrdal Station and what happened there.

After we talked about Flåm, Ron told me about a new camera he'd just bought. Ron and I often talked about cameras and photography whenever we bumped into one another. He had his new camera with him and showed me its tilting viewing screen. He thought it would be good for me because I had trouble moving and changing positions. Yes, I did need a new camera.

I've loved taking photos ever since Mum taught me how and gave me a Kodak Box Brownie as a child. I'd bought a few cameras since then. The one I was currently using was the one I'd taken on our last trip, to Egypt and Jordan in early 2010. It was a digital compact Nikon with a small zoom lens. There was a long lag time between pressing the button and the shutter releasing to take the photo. I had to remember to hold the camera steady during that time. There were quite a few blurred photos from that trip! My MS often made my hands clumsy, especially my left hand. I'd dropped that camera more than once.

When I had to resign from work in late 2006, the board of my organisation gave me a Canon 400D EOS digital SLR camera as a farewell gift. Although that was my first digital SLR, I did have a film SLR that I bought a long time ago. I went to Singapore to buy a Nikon F2 in the late 1970s because it was cheaper to buy it there than in Australia. The difference in price between Singapore and Australia paid for the airfare. Now I was thinking of cameras again.

The Canon 400D SLR was a beautiful camera, but it was too heavy for me to take travelling.

After talking with Ron and thinking about how much I love taking photos, I decided I really did want to buy a new camera to take on my trip to Norway.

When I was out on my scooter, it was sometimes hard to get close enough to what I wanted to photograph. So I looked at cameras with bigger zoom lenses. My current camera was a Nikon Coolpix 4800 with an 8.3x zoom. I'd had it for about six years and I'd also been reading about cameras with much bigger zoom lenses than that.

I had my eye on another Nikon Coolpix. It was the P100. It had a 26x optical zoom lens. The camera's zoom range was 26 to 678 millimetres in the old language of 35-millimetre film. That was an enormous range. I decided that was what I wanted.

Then I wondered how I'd go about getting the camera. In the past, I'd always gone to a large camera shop. I'd have a good look at the different options available. But it's not that easy for me to get to a camera shop any more. I began by checking prices online. An online vendor had the cheapest price by far. I hadn't bought anything like a camera online before. But I took the chance.

I was impressed with the service. I received emails confirming my order and letting me know the camera was on its way. Within a few days, there was a buzz at the door. My new camera was delivered. It had been very securely packaged and all was in working order!

The new camera with a 26x optical zoom lens came in mid-May. That was something else organised and ready to go for the trip.

In terms of the trip bookings, I just needed to finish off the transport around the Nutshell. I looked at Ron's excursion notes for trips in the Flåm area and they all said 'Not suitable for wheelchairs'. But I knew I could wait a bit a longer for further information that would be first-hand, with Ron and Carolyn's help. I could wait a bit longer.

Not long after I bought the new camera, Sue came home from golf one day with another idea. She thought we should discuss our travel plans with Raina. Sue had heard about Raina from one of her golf partners. Raina was originally from Norway but now she lived in Melbourne for part of the year and the rest of the year with family back in Norway. Raina should be able to help with our questions.

Sue telephoned Raina. We had our questions written out all ready to ask. Instead, Raina invited us to visit her, to discuss it in person. We arranged a time.

At about the same time as Sue was organising this, I received a phone call from my neurologist. He left a message on my mobile phone. 'Maureen, the JC Virus blood test was negative. The level is so low that it's regarded as not being present. So, that's good. Continue on with the Tysabri.'

Great news, I thought. Thank goodness! It meant that I knew my risk of getting PML was actually very very low, negligible even. I also thought that it was wonderful of him to phone me personally. I was going to see him soon anyway, for one of my routine six-monthly appointments.

I saw my neurologist on 25 May. I went up in the lift to see him in his rooms after my thirtieth Tysabri infusion. He was in the same building as the Day Chemotherapy Unit. I enjoyed seeing him and getting an update on how I was doing. I tried to have everything organised and to have copies of test results from my GP or other doctors ready to give him, in case they'd not been sent. I sometimes rehearsed what I had to remember to say in the days before the appointment.

I rode my new yellow Luggie scooter into his consultation room. He hadn't seen one before, so I explained it all to him. He seemed very impressed.

While I was seeing him, I was able to double-check the dates of my infusions and check what changes I might have to make.

The scheduled date for the infusion was 14 September, in the middle of the cruise. My neurologist said I could move the date to 28 September, and then receive the infusion every four weeks after that. I'd been on Tysabri for just over two years. It was okay to shift it those two weeks for this trip.

'How's your six-minute walk going?' he asked as he was reviewing my history.

'Good,' I said. 'It hasn't changed. I can still do eighteen laps on my walker around the kitchen bench in six minutes.' I had measured and calculated that distance to be about two hundred metres. I checked the time every few months.

'That's a four-wheel walker you use, isn't it?' he asked.

'Yes.'

'How long do you think you can walk with it now?'

'I can still walk for twenty minutes with the walker without stopping. But after that I can hardly move my legs and I need to stop, sit down and rest. I get slower too towards the end of the twenty minutes. I try to do that walk at least twice a week. Otherwise, I use my electric wheelchair when I'm getting about inside.'

'And when you walk with your walker outside, what distance would that cover?'

'I think it's about six hundred metres.'

'That's good.' And he wrote that down.

I could only do that distance and that duration about twice a week. It took hours to recover and sometimes a whole day. I knew it was important for me to exercise and I had a programme from the MS physiotherapist that I tried to follow religiously. I really believed that exercise was important. I've always enjoyed some form of exercise.

Then I added, 'Oh, and I leave the walker beside my bed at night and use it when I get up to go to the toilet.'

'How many times do you get up at night?'

'Twice, sometimes three times.'

'Do you want to see someone about that?'

'Not at the moment, thanks, it's all right. I go back to sleep straight away afterwards.'

I went on to tell him that I'd a melanoma removed from my toe in February. He already had a copy of the pathology report, and was pleased that the melanoma had only been at Level 1 and was completely excised. He also said that there'd been some talk about the increased incidence of melanoma in people on Tysabri. However, he thought that the incidence was the same as persons exposed to sunlight in their youth. I was still surprised by the location on the outer edge of my little toe but that didn't seem to worry him.

He thought I was doing well with my MS and on Tysabri. I was to continue with the infusions. We talked about my next overseas trip before I left.

'Norway, the Arctic, mmmm. Well, enjoy yourself. I'd like to see you again in six months.'

I made the next appointment for the same day of my infusion in six months' time.

We visited Raina in the last days of May. We bought her afternoon tea and drove to her place. We sat in her lounge room and chatted. Raina was well into her seventies. She explained how she always caught either the bus or the train from Oslo Airport into the city of Oslo. 'It's too expensive to go any other way. The bus is the cheapest. The train fares keep going up.'

She asked where we were staying in Oslo and I showed her the map with the apartment marked. 'Oh, that's just across from the park. You can get the bus to here or here. There are several stops. Then you just walk across the park.'

'Oh, thanks. I didn't realise a stop would be so close.'

I had in mind possibly catching the train from the airport to Oslo Central Station. From there, we could get a taxi to the apartment. It would be very early in the morning, about 6 a.m. The bus was another option, I now realised. I asked Raina about taking my wheelchair-scooter on to the bus, but she didn't know.

We asked Raina what were the main things we just had to see in Oslo and in Bergen. Raina gave us a short list for each main city. In Oslo, she said we should see:

- The Viking Ship Museum, by ferry
- The sculpture park, walking
- The ski jump

In Bergen, Raina said we should see:

- The funicular
- Grieg's home
- The shops on the wharf, Bryggen

We talked about buying food and wine. 'Vinmonopolet,' Raina quickly jumped in. 'It's the government-controlled liquor store. It's wonderful. There's a great variety there, even Australian wines like Jacob's Creek.'

What to wear? Raina said, 'Mittens not gloves and a hat with ears.'

I asked about the Nutshell, but Raina couldn't give me much information about it. However, the list of places to go and Vinmonopolet sounded like wonderful advice.

About five weeks after we'd spoken with them in the car park, Ron and Sandra, true to their word, sent me an email with photos of the trains at Myrdal Station. That was sometime in early June. The two trains to change between were on either side of the same platform, at the same station. Easy.

Carolyn was in Norway from 8–20 June. She was doing the Nutshell part first, on the way from Oslo to Bergen, and then doing the coastal cruise. She sent several email messages. There were some just to say hello and let us know they were all having a great time. She was also checking out one of the places where we were staying.

Then Carolyn sent an SMS with some urgency. 'I have just been to the hotel that you booked in Flåm. The manager showed me your room. It is on the ground floor but it looks right on to the car park. There is a better room with a view and a nice balcony on the second floor. There is a lift. Do I have your permission to change the room number?'

'Yes, thank you. I didn't realise that there was a lift.' I had asked all the other accessibility questions. But from the advice I was given in the email from the tourist office, about being able to book a ground-floor room, I just assumed there were no lifts. I saw the photo of the hotel when doing the booking online. It had three levels. I assumed incorrectly that there were only stairs between them. Carolyn took several photos of the room, the view and the bathroom and sent them. That new room looked fantastic.

Carolyn and her friends had come down the Flåm Line from Myrdal after leaving Oslo. Carolyn sent an email to say she'd taken photos of the train at Myrdal and would show us those on her return. After checking the hotel in Flåm, Carolyn caught the ferry to Gudvangen. She took photos of the ferry too. She said it wasn't easy, but it was possible for me to do it.

As well as the NSB booking service, I'd also been able to access the ferry booking schedules in the fjords using the Fjord1 website. I could work out the times with changeovers on my own now. I could book the ferry trips straight away but the trains could only be booked within ninety days of departure. I still had to wait a little bit longer to do that.

It was June, the frenzied golf competition season had finished and it was winter in Melbourne. Sue and I had both been busy and it was time for a trip north to Queensland again.

CHAPTER 3
AIRPORTS AND TRAMS

I like airports for all the obvious reasons. They mean I'm going to get on a plane and fly somewhere. I like them especially if the plane is flying a very long way away and mostly if the plane is going outside Australia. Going to the airport to go overseas is always the most exciting.

But the largest numbers of flights I've taken have been domestic ones. My first flight was from Sydney to Melbourne when I was about thirteen years old. I went on my own. My friends and their parents picked me up at the airport and I went to stay with them in the country town of Shepparton.

My first overseas trip was to New Zealand with my parents and younger brothers when I was fifteen years old. It was in winter. The family business, where we all worked, closed down in winter. Mum ran a guesthouse at the time, with 'full board' for up to one hundred guests. People came there only in the warmer months. While we were in New Zealand, we were lucky enough to go on a light aircraft from Milford Sound to somewhere near the Franz Josef Glacier. We landed on the glacier and that was very exciting. I've always loved window seats and views. My love of them could have started then. The scenery through that window was spectacular.

For a while, I commuted between Sydney and Brisbane every week. Throughout my working life, I had a holiday once a year, overseas whenever I could afford it. Airports had just become a process to go through, with occasional extra waiting and queuing. I didn't think much about it. Being in the air and being where the plane landed was what it was all about.

My routine at airports suddenly changed as soon as I developed MS. I couldn't walk without something and someone to help me. Airports became a whole new place. Things that had never crossed my mind were now a series of sagas to go through.

Although my yellow scooter was getting a lot of experience with domestic flights, I was keen to iron out any difficulties that might arise before we left to go to Norway and the Arctic.

Each time I'd travelled with it, some part of the airport process was different. And that was just within Australia. For our flight north in June, we were going directly from Melbourne to the Sunshine Coast (Maroochydore) on a flight with Jetstar.

My series of new airport sagas began with getting there. In Melbourne, a taxi was best. I'd recently changed from calling a general taxi company to using a small taxi firm. Alan, who ran the business, had learned about my mobility equipment. There was enough space in his ordinary sedan cars to fit my scooter. He told his drivers that it wasn't much trouble to lift it into the boot. Sue usually helped them too.

Some taxis in the past, at the taxi rank, had refused to take me when they saw me on the scooter (or the wheelchair before it). They shook their heads and left without waiting for any explanation of how the device collapsed and how it easily fitted into most taxi boots. Some drivers had refused to help Sue lift the scooter into the boot. It did need one or two people to lift it over the lip of a sedan boot. Sometimes, I was the one who helped Sue lift it in.

For the trip in June, I'd ordered a taxi with Alan a few days before by SMS. The taxi arrived on time and parked directly outside the entrance to our apartment block. I rode the scooter through the doorway. We collapsed it down and I walked with my stick and Sue's arm to the already open front taxi door. It was much easier for me to get into the front passenger side than into the back. There was more room for lifting my legs in.

The driver was pleasant and helpful. The scooter went into the boot easily and the cab was lovely and clean inside. We were at the airport in twenty minutes.

We arrived at Melbourne Tullamarine Airport well ahead of schedule. As usual, the airline instructions said to be there at least one hour before the scheduled departure time. We had to allow plenty of time for the scooter to be booked in and to find a wheelchair for my wheelchair-assistance booking. The taxi stopped right outside the Jetstar entrance at T1 Domestic.

I signed the form for the Victorian Taxi Directorate, Multi Purpose Taxi Programme and paid in cash for my half of the fare, with a tip for the driver. This was a wonderful scheme for people living in Victoria, provided by the Victorian government's Department of Transport. The programme was for people using wheelchairs who required taxi transport. I only had to pay for half the fare. The government paid the taxi service the other half and Alan's taxis were happy to take the card (unlike some others in the past).

The taxi driver opened the boot and Sue helped him get my scooter out. She assembled it ready to go. I got out with my walking stick and put my handbag around my neck. The driver got out our one luggage bag. Sue had her backpack on and her handbag over her shoulder. She put the computer bag on my lap. We thanked the driver, waved him off and moved inside the terminal, with Sue wheeling the luggage bag.

The Jetstar check-in area had a line of people queued up. Sue and I joined the queue, with me on my scooter. An airline attendant, wearing the Jetstar black and orange colours, came up to us and said, 'Where are you going?'

'Maroochydore,' I said. 'The Sunshine Coast.'

The Jetstar attendant opened a barrier cord and directed us to another area in front of the check-in counters with no queue. That was a bonus. Sometimes, at airports, I'd just queue up with everyone else and wind around and around the cordoned passageway. Sometimes Sue would go and find an attendant and ask if we needed to do anything special, hoping to be placed on another queue. Getting to the check-in counter was going to be much easier today, I thought.

After a few minutes, it was our turn to be called forward. When the check-in person, a young woman, looked up, she gave us a frightened look. People don't usually look so frightened when they see me at check-in counters. I scooted forward, reached up and gave the young woman my little pile of paperwork for the booking and the scooter. The booking itinerary, printed out for the two of us, was on the top, together with my ID. Sue was behind me getting her ID out. 'Have you booked a wheelchair?'

'Yes, I have,' I answered, thinking that there was a symbol of a wheelchair beside my name, under 'Extras' on the booking sheet in front of her. I'd done the right thing.

'Are you taking that with you?' she asked looking at the scooter.

'Yes, I am,' I replied.

'You look really worried,' Sue said to her.

'I'm not worried. I just haven't done one of these before. I'll have to go and ask a supervisor. I think I need to fill out a form.' The young woman left the counter and returned with some papers and an older woman, who took over the questioning.

'Hello. What kind of a battery does it have?'

'Lithium,' I answered. She looked at the young woman, nodding at the paperwork, and then at me again.

'You look like you've done this before.'

'Yes, I have.' We all smiled at each other. We were all nodding our heads by then.

The lithium battery was different to the gel cell battery that I'd had before for the blue wheelchair. Although they were both dry cell batteries (rather than wet cell), the lithium battery was made of lithium ion and was a potentially explosive substance. I'd learned the hard way that I needed to do a few extra things when flying with it.

The first time I flew with the scooter, I went to the check-in desk without any paperwork for it. After initially being told that I wasn't allowed to put the scooter on board as baggage, somehow, after a lot of checking, phoning, looking at the battery, discussion and jumping up and down in protest, they allowed it.

Travelling with a lithium ion battery larger than one in a digital camera or a laptop was new for everyone, it seemed. The writing on the back of my battery read that it had a rating of 220 Wh. That first time, I had no paperwork to say it was safe. I didn't know that I needed dangerous-goods approval. I didn't know that I had to show and travel with a copy of the material safety data sheet (MSDS) for the battery. There were special regulations for lithium ion batteries – for their size, removal, storage and the protective covering of any exposed terminals. I had no idea. The gel cell battery was different and had its own simpler regulations.

There was a limit to the number of 'Wh' allowed for a lithium ion battery. I had to look that up. Originally, when I saw 'Wh', I thought it was a typo and that it meant 'watts'. But when I looked it up, I realised 'Wh' was short for 'watt-hours'. It was an energy measurement, not a power measurement, and the number really mattered. I was fascinated by it all for a while. I also obtained a MSDS from the supplier as fast as I could.

'We need the approval number,' the older woman said to the younger one.

'Did you get approval?' she asked me.

'Yes, I telephoned through as soon as I did the booking online.' There was a two-way radio call and a conversation between the older woman and someone else on the line.

I pointed out the MSDS front page, which was in a plastic cover-sheet with the paperwork I'd handed in. The document's other five pages were attached. 'Gee, you are well-organised.' Yes, I thought, I'd learned. I smiled and nodded.

The person at the other end of the two-way radio call gave a number and the younger woman wrote it down on her paperwork.

'How much does the scooter weigh? Around about?' asked the older woman.

'Twenty-three kilograms.'

'How many bags?' asked the younger woman.

'Just one,' said Sue. 'And with the scooter, that's two luggage tags.' Sue put our bag on to the conveyor belt and noted that it weighed twelve kilograms. We needed to carry even less than usual for this trip to a warmer climate.

The young woman put a baggage tag around the suitcase. She handed the other baggage tag to the older woman, who asked, 'Where do they usually put this?' I turned around and pointed to the bar that ran at the back of the scooter. There were marks on it from bits of old tags from previous trips.

'Do you want to take it to the gate or do you want a wheelchair from here and we'll take it now?'

'I'd like to take it to the gate, please.'

Sue jumped in and said, 'But there has to be a wheelchair at the gate when you take the scooter.' As Sue said this, we both remembered those times when there'd been no wheelchair and they'd asked me if I could walk along the passageway to the air bridge or walk out on to the tarmac to the lifter. No, I need a wheelchair, please, I said every time.

'Yes, there'll be a wheelchair there. Are you able to walk up the stairs or do you need a lifter?'

Jetstar was a budget airline, an offshoot of Qantas Airlines. They didn't have air-bridge links from inside the terminal to the aircraft door at Melbourne Airport. The Jetstar planes used the far ends of the terminal where passengers walked outside along the tarmac to get to the plane and then ascended a set of steps. The same thing applied at most smaller airports, such as where we were going that day.

'No, I can't walk up that many steps. I need the lifter, please.' The young woman finished ticking the boxes on the form and handed the papers to me.

'You need to give them this paperwork at the gate. You must be there thirty minutes before departure – that's 9.30 a.m.' The younger woman handed me our boarding passes and I checked the seats that she had allocated. They were 4B and 4C. I showed Sue.

Sue asked 'Is it a full flight? If we sit in those seats, Maureen has to get up to let someone out. I know that one has to be on the aisle and that's an airline requirement, but…'

'It's not a full flight and I've blocked the other seat so you can have the full row.'

'Thank you, that's terrific.' Great, I thought. I could have a window seat and look out. Otherwise, they wouldn't give me a window seat, even if I booked one and paid for it online beforehand.

'Okay, thanks again,' we both said and we were off.

We went to the boarding gates where there were lines of people queuing to go through the security checkpoints. I looked for a sign with a wheelchair symbol and cardiac pacemaker reference on it. The two things usually went together. Sue and I both saw the sign and joined the queue there.

There were five lines. But it seemed there was only one line at an area at the end, which allowed people to move through without going through the detector. They went around the detector through a gate if they were in a wheelchair or if they had a pacemaker inserted, like my mother.

When we were putting our bags and things into plastic containers to go through the security machines, a man in a security uniform came over and said, 'You have to go over there,' and pointed to another line. There was no sign to see but the man directed us to move to that line anyway. I didn't question what line it was. I just did what I was told. We went straight over and a nice man (he looked like a Chinese tourist) let us go in front of him. We didn't have to join another queue and I could see there was an area at the end around the detector.

I put my walking stick into the plastic container with my handbag. I unlatched the scooter carry bag, attached to the back of the seat, took it off and put it on the conveyor belt too. Sue pulled the computer out of its bag and placed that in another plastic container with her handbag, and put her backpack in another one. Sue's backpack contained the scooter's charging unit and our travel documents.

Sue walked through the detector and collected all our bits

and pieces together. She repeated a number to herself as she went through to remind herself how many items to pick up at the end. Neither of us wanted to lose any of them.

I went around the detector and through the plastic gates that the security people opened. I was signalled to a rubber mat and stopped at the point I was told. A woman in uniform came up to me and said, 'I'm going to give you a security check. Are you familiar with that? Is that okay with you?'

'Yes, fine.' The woman proceeded to pat me down as I lifted and spread my arms out. Another woman came over and ran some sort of handheld detector over the scooter to check it too.

I met Sue once I was through and put my walking stick back in place on my scooter and Sue attached the carry bag to the back of my seat. The computer bag was on my lap and Sue had the backpack and handbags. She handed me my handbag and we were set to go. We were doing well time-wise to get to Gate 30, way down at the end of the terminal.

We went to the right and then around a corner to get to a lift. We went down one level (half a floor) and then went out and around, to get on to the straight path leading to Gates 21 to 30. At the end, near Gate 30, there was another small lift to go down one floor. There were so many lifts in the terminal, all in hidden places it seemed. I'd worked them all out by then. When I was first in a wheelchair at an airport, it took a bit of time to find them. At least there were lifts in Melbourne. At least they were usually working.

At Gate 30, we went up to the counter and handed the paperwork from check-in to the Jetstar attendant. The attendant made a call on her two-way radio for a baggage handler. Sue asked for a wheelchair and the attendant brought one over, telling us that we'd be boarding first. She looked at us carefully and then walked off without saying anything, leaving us to organise the scooter.

I got off the scooter and had a stretch. I took out the battery and gave it to Sue. Sue got the canvas bag out of the carry bag on the back of scooter seat and handed me a strip of polystyrene from inside. I'd turned the polystyrene, which I'd got from some packing inside a parcel, into an insulation strip. I put it over the exposed battery terminal connections on the scooter. Sue put the battery in bubble wrap and then into the canvas carry bag. I undid the clamps holding the tiller up so that it could collapse down to the lowest level. Then I pulled the lever on the tiller's side to make it go completely flat down on the scooter and fastened it in place with the clip. I finally sat on the airline wheelchair. My jobs were finished.

Sue got an old bag covering with a clip tie out of the canvas bag. The old bag covering was a black polypropylene shopping bag turned inside out to hide the store's labeling, which allowed me to put on my own labels. I'd photographed and then printed two signs on A4 canvas photo paper. One was a disability wheelchair sign and the other was a 'Fragile' sign from an old paper airline tag. I'd sewn the canvas labels on to the blank side of the old black bag.

Sue put the old bag over the back of the seat and tied the handles together in the space underneath, before folding the back down forward on to the seat. Then she squeezed the piece at the base of the scooter to release the seat and collapsed it down flat too. With everything collapsed down, the labels were clear to see. We hoped that seeing the labels might help make the baggage handlers treat my precious scooter gently. We always crossed our fingers!

After collapsing the scooter down with the bag on, Sue put a long clip tie around the middle of the width of scooter and over the top of the seat to hold it all firmly together.

The baggage handler arrived dressed in his grey overalls and earmuffs. Sue showed him the best way to wheel the scooter to move it and undid the wheel lock. He took the scooter away. I always thought at that point in the airline sequence of events that I hoped I'd see it again at the other end.

I once lost my old blue wheelchair on a Los Angeles to Honolulu transfer in 2007. The airline delivered it to the hotel the next day, with its pieces together but not attached like they were before. Despite that, the bits went back together and it still worked well. The airline also lent me a big manual wheelchair to use in the meantime. Well, it was more that Sue had demanded the wheelchair, seeing as they lost mine! And then she'd had to push that with me in it, as well as pull our bag. It wasn't easy but we had more people around then who could help.

We sat at Gate 30 and waited for the call. There were two other people in wheelchairs. The attendant came over and asked Sue if she was able to push me part of the way. The attendant explained, 'We only have one staff member on to take the wheelchairs out today.' Oh, I thought, now I'm a wheelchair, not a person!

Sometimes people talk to Sue and ignore me. I think, Hello! I'm here! I can listen, understand and talk too.

The boarding sign lit up on the screen over the gateway and the airline attendant led the way. We went out down a covered passageway. The attendant went first, pushing one wheelchair, and Sue followed with me. We stopped where the covering ended and we were on the edge of the open tarmac. It was very windy and cold. The attendant left to collect the other person in a wheelchair. Soon all three of us 'wheelchairs' were parked there. I think the airline policy changed some time after that, allowing only two people who required wheelchairs to be booked on the same flight.

I waited my turn for the attendant to take me to the lifter. 'Are you able to stand in the lifter?' she asked.

'Yes, I can.' In the distance, two men wheeled out the large lifting device and placed it adjacent to the steps leading up to the front door of the aircraft. The lifting part had a flat platform with a semicircle of metal rising up from the base. The metal circle went three quarters of the way around, up to chest level. The metal surround was open at one end, just wide enough to fit either a person walking in or a wheelchair wheeled in. Inside, it could fit one person in a wheelchair with an attendant or two people standing with one attendant. There was a clear plastic waterproof cover over the top and at the sides, in case it rained. A man driving a forklift came over to lift it up.

Sue walked over the tarmac and up the steps into the aircraft. The attendant wheeled me to the lifter. I stepped out of the wheelchair with my walking stick and held her arm. I stepped into the lifter and hung on to the metal handrail running around it. The attendant came in after me and then signalled to the forklift driver. The lifter rose up towards the top of the stairs that led into the airplane's entry door. There was a platform at the top of the stairs and that also extended out to one side. The extension had a gate at the edge. The lifter moved up and down, backwards and forwards a few times before it was level with the gate and the platform. A few times, I had to grab on tightly to the thin metal handrail. Once we were all level, the attendant opened the gate and directed me out, offering her arm to help me get across the platform.

When we flew into Ushuaia, at the very bottom of South America, to go to Antarctica, two men carried me down the stairs. I was sitting in an airline wheelchair because, as well as no air bridge, they had no lifter. But how wonderful it was for them to give me such personal service. I didn't even think to ask ahead of time. I just assumed that if I'd booked a wheelchair that the link between the plane and the terminal would be there. Well, I suppose it was!

It was an easy, short and level walk from the lifter to the aircraft door, where there was just one low step to go up and in. I bent over and used my left hand behind my knee to lift my left leg up, leaning with my stick and right hand against the door. I was soon in and the cabin attendant greeted me.

'Hello, my name is Carl. I'll be your cabin manager today. What seat are you in? Do you need help to get there?'

'Hello, it's 4C and I can walk using my stick and the top of the seats, thank you.' Carl waited until I reached the fourth row of seats. Sue was already waiting there too. She had put the backpack up in the storage area and was waiting to put my walking stick up there as well. Sue let me get in first to 4B so that I could move over to the 4A window seat.

The cabin manager waited until I was sitting in my seat and then explained the emergency safety procedures to us. After he finished he said, 'If you need any other assistance or have any questions, we're here. Just press this button.'

Then he came back. 'Oh, and when we arrive, if you could wait to get off last, please. Do you need a wheelchair at the other end too?'

'Sure, and, yes, I do, please.'

'I'll call ahead and let them know.'

'Thank you.'

With all those steps completed, finally sitting in the plane, I've always had a mix of feelings. A sense of relief that all that getting into the aircraft is over and that I'm about to fly away somewhere. The last-minute adrenalin rush from trying to remember everything, closing the door at home and getting out to the airport on time had passed. If we'd forgotten to pack anything, it didn't matter any more. We'd either buy a substitute or just cope.

I organised my reading glasses and book for when we were up in the air. I sat there looking out of the window and feeling good. Then there was that wonderful feeling when the plane takes off, with my eyes slowly closing and then opening again, seconds or many minutes later, to find myself in another world.

Once we were up in the air and cruising, the captain made an announcement welcoming people on board. He said, 'Today we'll be flying over Wagga Wagga, heading north and going just east of Dubbo, on to the Gold Coast and then on to Maroochydore. The weather for our arrival should be a warm and sunny twenty-three degrees.'

The flight time was about two hours. I read and then, after about an hour or so, I felt my legs becoming stiff. I was moving my feet and legs every few minutes, but they still felt stiff. I told Sue and she said, 'I want to go to the toilet anyway, so you can get up and stretch. Do you want to go to the toilet too?'

'No, I'll wait, but I'll get up and stretch.' I followed Sue out of the seat into the aisle. It was an aircraft with about thirty rows and two hundred passengers, configured three by three. Sue walked on to the toilet. I stood in the aisle and started to do an exercise that my MS physiotherapist had shown me. She'd told me that, whenever I got a chance, this was a good exercise to do for my legs and balance.

It was a subtle and inconspicuous movement so I thought I'd do it while I was standing in the aisle. I was facing the front of the aircraft. The exercise involved moving my legs by slowly bending and straightening my knees slightly and alternately while keeping my feet together. I counted to myself as I did it.

After a few minutes, the cabin attendant came up to me from the rear of the plane and said, 'There's another toilet down the back, if you want to use that.'

'Oh, thank you, but I'm just moving my legs for a bit of exercise.' Oh dear, I thought, I suppose it looked as though I was trying to hang on from wanting to go to the toilet. Some people in the rows of people behind me were probably watching and thinking the same thing. I stopped moving and just stood in the aisle for a while, holding on to the top of the seats. I didn't want to go to the toilet yet.

Sometimes the distance between the top of a seat, which I could hold on to, and the toilet door was too far to walk, especially on a bumpy ride. Sue or an attendant would have to give me an arm to lean on. Sometimes where my seat was on the plane was very important.

Sue came back and I'd finished stretching and felt better, so we both took our seats. Through the window, I could see the Tweed Valley as we headed over to the Gold Coast. After going over the canal housing developments and the high-rise buildings along the beach, the plane flew up the coastline. We went over South Stradbroke Island, North Stradbroke Island and Moreton Island. Moreton Bay spread out to the west with the Brisbane city skyline not far up along the Brisbane River.

The colour of the water was a brilliant turquoise and I could see patterns in the sand where the water wasn't deep. Moreton Bay was beautiful, and sometimes the scenes from the air looked like works of art spread out on a canvas. Looking out at scenes like that reminded me of why I loved flying and loved window seats.

We headed out to sea and I followed the coastline north as we flew over Bribie Island. The Sunshine Coast soon followed. I had the map pictured in my mind and saw all the towns: Caloundra,

Alexandra Headland, Maloolaba and Maroochydore. In my mind, I was melding the actual place and the location on the map into one. I could see the map clearly. At times, I wonder if I have a kind of photographic memory.

As we approached our destination, we flew low over Twin Waters and its golf course. Sue and Carolyn had played golf there one time and I went around with them on my Parmaker three-wheel heavy-duty outdoor scooter. It was a lovely course with lots of trees, and sometimes there were kangaroos on the greens. That grey Parmaker was the first scooter I'd bought. I'd wanted something that I could use on walking tracks, golf courses and other rough terrain. I had trouble walking long distances then and wanted to be able to get out and about in natural surroundings and do some outdoor activities. I even went up and over the edge of the volcanic rim into Wilpena Pound on a holiday in South Australia. It wasn't a conventional mobility scooter.

Maroochydore Airport was the main airport for the Sunshine Coast in Queensland. We were last off. The process after that was mostly the same as boarding, just in reverse.

It was a small airport. There were no air bridges, just stairs on wheels and lifters on wheels with forklifts. Everything was the same as always except for my scooter. Sue waited for me to come out of the lifter and then the attendant handed the wheelchair over to Sue to push. We found our way, following the signs to the baggage collection area.

Our bag usually came out on the conveyor belt with everyone else's, and the scooter usually came out at a 'special luggage' or an 'oversized luggage' area. In the past, my wheelchair or the scooter had come out on the moving conveyor belt, sometimes upside down. I could see it was very difficult for Sue to lift thirty kilograms of blue wheelchair or twenty-three kilograms of yellow scooter as it moved along the conveyer belt. That wasn't supposed to happen.

At Maroochydore, the bag arrived first and Sue deposited it beside me. She went off to find the scooter, wheeled it over to where I was sitting, untied the clip tie, and then, squeezing the catch at the base, lifted the seat up and into place ready for use. I just stepped out of the wheelchair and on to the scooter. Sue moved the wheelchair out of the way, and off we went.

I'd booked a rental car for us to pick up at Maroochydore Airport. We went over to the Avis counter and presented our booking paperwork. Thankfully, the AWD wagon was available and we made our way outside to the car, finished with an airport for a little while.

My series of airport sagas that began with leaving home and getting to the airport was followed by so many more afterwards. Now, having so many parts to the process – getting to, on and off a plane – I wonder how I ever travelled before without noticing them. I didn't think anything much about it at all before my mobility was affected. I just went to the airport and boarded a plane!

I have a list of the steps I need to go through just to get inside the plane and there were more after that. At every one of those steps, I'd learned there were a number of different scenarios that might happen. Any step could turn into an adventure.

1. Getting to the airport
2. Getting to the check-in counter
3. At check-in
4. Leaving check-in on my scooter or in a wheelchair
5. Going through security first or after the next step
6. Getting to passport and immigration control
7. Going through passport and immigration control
8. Getting to the boarding gate
9. At the boarding gate
10. Getting to the aircraft
11. Boarding the aircraft
12. Inside the aircraft

Each of the steps, on the list and to follow, has involved some sort of story, all of its own. Sue and I had to laugh about it afterwards. 'What about the time…?' Many of the most interesting stories came from the steps after we landed.

On our trip to Egypt, we landed at Cairo Airport and my blue electric wheelchair was brought out to me fully assembled, not as we'd packed it. It looked okay at first glance but when I went outside and tried to turn in it, it went around in circles. By then, it was too late to go back inside, and it was Cairo – bustling and very foreign. We just scrambled into a small tour bus and went to the hotel.

Luckily, when we told our story at the reception desk we found out that there was a hotel maintenance area and they had someone working there who'd try to help. He came to our room with our guide and looked at the wheelchair. We turned it upside down and on its side to find that one of the heavy metal pieces connected to the light aluminium was very bent. He took the wobbly chair away to his workroom and straightened out the metal again.

I realised what had happened when we were departing Cairo on the next flight to Luxor. At check-in, they were loading the wheelchair with the baggage on to conveyor belts that turned 90° on their way to the loading area. I saw some bags get stuck and could imagine the wheelchair at 90° being bent towards 180°. 'No, no,' I said. 'The wheelchair cannot go along there with the bags.'

Sue said, 'It has to go as "special luggage". You do have special luggage, don't you?' There were blank looks.

'Where do you put fragile things, like big pieces of glass or crockery or things like that? Things that might break,' asked Sue. There were still blank looks. We looked to our guide for help.

"They don't have special baggage,' he said.

'Oh, okay. What about heavy luggage or things that are not bags, where do they go? It can't go on the luggage belt. Someone or some people will have to carry it to be loaded.' We tried to explain. The guide translated what we said into Arabic and soon two men came out to collect the wheelchair. I hope I see it again, I thought. It did arrive at the end of the flight and it wasn't bent. But we had to go through the same performance at each airport after that, in both Egypt and Jordan.

I felt that I'd become quite experienced and, after a while, I didn't notice anything that was just 'the usual' any more. Whatever happened just happened. The vast majority of the time, for most of the flying process and the airport sagas, there was nothing that was really different in the process. When something happened that was different or stood out for some reason, I really did notice it. For me, flights had become a bit as they used to be, except now it was just going through a familiar 'airport process' and boarding a plane. I still liked airports, because, in the end, they still meant the same thing. It was just a bit different now. I didn't look at the list again after I'd made it!

The only part of the airport process that remained unfamiliar was travelling with my new yellow scooter and its lithium battery on international flights.

On that day, flying to the Sunshine Coast, all went well and there were no stories of any note to tell or even think about writing of afterwards. It was all just the usual airport process.

While we were up there, we went shopping at Sunshine Plaza in Maroochydore. I liked going to that shopping centre because everywhere was accessible. It was easy to go into shops because the entries were level with the outside passageways – no lips or steps to get over. The shopping centre also had working lifts and disabled toilets together with air conditioning (a great relief when it became very hot in Queensland). Shopping there was easy.

***

I bought my first walking stick in a shopping centre. It wasn't at the Sunshine Plaza or anywhere else in Queensland. It was in NSW, at Chatswood, on a Sunday, at a large shopping centre called Chatswood Chase. Up until that particular Sunday, it had been easy for me to occasionally walk around the centre and shop. I only came to understand years later that on that day I was at the beginning of an episode of MS, very early in the progressive phase.

To my surprise, I was having trouble walking along the flat floor. I felt terrible. I was on my own and thought, how am I going to get where I want to go? I was at the centre to buy something important

– a gift, perhaps. I felt as if I was about to fall over at any minute. What was wrong? It must be related to the fall I had when I was bushwalking yesterday, I thought. When that happened, I couldn't lift my leg for a while back in the car. My left leg seemed okay now. I planned to make an appointment to see a neurologist during the next week. It'll be okay till then, I thought.

But I had to do something right then and there. I need a walking stick, I told myself. I think I'll feel better with one. I needed something to hold on to. I'll go and buy one right away, I said to myself. Where do I buy a walking stick? A pharmacy, of course. There must be one in the shopping centre.

I didn't have to look too far before I saw a pharmacy. I went in and asked the shop assistant if they had any walking sticks. Yes, they did, and she showed me to the section. 'We only have one left' she said. 'This cane one with a round handle.' I tried it and it seemed okay. Despite my medical training, I knew nothing about the correct height for a walking stick, what side to use it on or how to use it. None of these things even occurred to me at the time.

The cane stick did seem okay, so I bought it. As soon as I started to use it, I felt so much better. I didn't feel off-balance any more and I felt supported. There was also less effort required to move along. I felt confident about walking again. So I continued shopping, walking with my new walking stick.

Then I thought – are people looking at me? I didn't look old or feeble. I looked young and strong, I thought. People would surely be looking at me and thinking I was odd. I briefly looked around as I walked along. No one was looking.

I've bought many more walking sticks since then. I don't look around to see if anyone is watching any more.

***

In the Sunshine Plaza shopping centre in Queensland, on my yellow scooter with my walking stick folded and tucked into its base, I scooted past a stall in between the shops selling mobile phones. It really drew my attention. I had to stop.

I had my Nokia mobile phone and I didn't need anything else, I thought. But so many people had told me that I'd just love an iPhone if I had one. Pam, an old friend from Sydney, had said, 'It'll change your life. It would be great when you're travelling and you love those techno kind of things.' There in front of me was an opportunity to get one of these new high-tech phones.

The young man behind the counter was very helpful. I talked with him for some time and then went away with all sorts of notes, brochures and figures on the back of a business card. I said I'd like to think about it overnight. I'd think and talk it through back at the house, after a rest, I thought. There seemed a lot to consider and I needed to lie down anyway. It was by now late in the afternoon.

I needed to have a rest every day by late afternoon. A fatigue would come over me and I just had to lie my body down. My thoughts could become confused when I felt tired and they'd become clear again after a rest. Twenty minutes would usually do.

With a clearer mind after my rest, I thought about a new smartphone again. Initially, it seemed like it might be a bit expensive. The penny dropped when I realised I could use an iPhone to provide mobile internet access to my computer by turning on the phone's personal hotspot. I could replace my existing mobile internet card and plan, and my old mobile phone with my smartphone, and it would all add up to the same cost. And I'd have a new iPhone as well.

The next day I went back and bought an iPhone 4, my first smartphone. I signed up for a package deal with Telstra and cancelled the use of my other device. My new phone did everything I could do before and a whole a lot more. And it was a lot faster and more convenient. It opened up a whole new world for me.

I fell in love with my smartphone and was especially keen to master it before I travelled. I wanted to learn how to send emails at free Wi-Fi spots and to take photos to send with them. I wanted to be able to look things up on Google.

A few days after I bought my new phone, we flew back to

Melbourne so I could have my next Tysabri infusion. Those flights were cheap advance booking specials for AUD$69 per person each way. I'd jumped on to the website as soon as I received an alert months earlier and made several bookings.

All went well with the airport process on our way back until we picked up the scooter at Melbourne Airport. The yellow scooter arrived at special baggage looking normal, but when I sat down and straightened my back it tipped backwards. The securing clips halfway along the base were broken on both sides. We went to the nearest counter for our airline and reported it straight away. The Jetstar supervisor came out quickly and we explained what had happened and gave a demonstration. 'Oh, yes, I can see,' she said. 'Here's my phone number and take this reference number too.'

'Thank you,' I said as she handed me the piece of paper.

'Do you know someone who can repair it, a supplier or someone qualified?'

'Yes, the company from whom I bought the scooter should be able to fix it. They have a workshop attached to their showroom.'

'Good. Will you be able to get home with it now?'

'Yes, if I'm careful and keep straight we should be able to get out to the taxi.' I had one of Alan's organised to meet us.

'So, when you get home, ring the company and tell them that Jetstar will pay for the cost to repair it. You can either send the invoice directly to Jetstar or you can pay and then send the paperwork to Jetstar and they'll reimburse you. I'll write down the address for posting.'

'Wow, that's wonderful,' I said. 'Thank you.' I was so overcome with her helpfulness that I didn't get a chance to be annoyed.

Sue and I left, very impressed with the service we received from Jetstar. The scooter was, however, broken and we had to spend time getting it fixed. I needed my scooter for my outings and I also needed it to be ready for the trip ahead in just over three months' time. I didn't think it would be a major problem; it would only take an hour or so to fix and the Pollyanna in me also thought it was good that this happened because I could get a maintenance check done at the same time. That would be a good thing to have done before we left. The scooter had already had a lot of use in the eight months since I'd bought it.

I had my Tysabri infusion on 22 June and, shortly afterwards, my old friend Jan from university came down from Canberra to stay for a few days. It was great to see her again and we went to see the King Tut exhibition that was on at Melbourne Museum. My trip to Egypt had left me with an even greater fascination for all things Egyptian. King Tut's fabulous burial mask was part of the exhibition. I could get close to it in Melbourne, without the enormous crowds in the Egyptian museum. All that gold on it was incredible, and the blue lapis lazuli make-up was one of the most beautiful colours in the world.

Even with all those distractions, every now and then I would go on to the NSB website and look at train timetables. I wanted to check and double-check different ideas that I had. I still had to wait, though, for the timetable with the actual times to appear for the days I wanted.

By the end of June, the timetable was out. I could finally see the times for that third week of September. I was then within the ninety-day booking period and I knew the times to book. But I still wasn't sure how we'd get back to Flåm for the night. I wasn't going to book the trains until I'd figured it out.

Then July just happened and Carolyn was back. We met up and went through all the information she'd collected from Norway. Carolyn had maps, timetables, the Hurtigruten excursions brochure and lots of other bits and pieces of useful information that she'd collected along the way. She'd printed off my email and highlighted the important parts of my questions. She had answers for all of them, backed up with photos and much more to tell me.

Carolyn explained arriving at Oslo Airport first. She told me about the fast-train link. 'It's right there. At Oslo Airport, you just come out of arrivals, look to your right and it's there.' Carolyn went on to tell me, 'The train from the airport to the city was so easy. The carriage looked like you could just go straight in with your scooter.'

Then she told me about Myrdal Station and the short route across the platform to board the Flåm train that left from the other side. It was right there and easy. The hotel in Flåm was very close to where the Flåm Line route ended.

But even with all that Carolyn told me, I still wasn't sure how we'd get back to Flåm from Gudvangen. I reminded myself again that it was just those Nutshell bookings that were yet to do and, importantly, I still needed to book the train back to Oslo to get home. As tempting as it was to just book something, I couldn't do it. I wanted to do all those Nutshell bookings at the same time to make sure they'd all link in together. I wanted to wait until I felt absolutely confident.

I felt like one of the women in Chekov's play *Three Sisters*. I'll never forget seeing that play. I felt so infuriated by one of the sisters, who kept saying she was 'going to Moscow'. It drove me bananas! I was about to stand up in the middle of the theatre and yell out, 'Just go to Moscow! For goodness' sake, just go! Just do it.' I was thinking, please stop saying you're going to do something and then not do it! Then I remembered where I was. I can't recall why the sister couldn't or wouldn't go; maybe it was just a dream of hers. Regardless, I thought I had better reasons to leave those bookings for now. I couldn't 'just do it' yet. And I wasn't dreaming.

Before travelling overseas, I needed to see my GP. She had a practice in the city on Collins Street. I usually saw her about every four months and went there by tram. I enjoy catching the tram. In some ways, it's similar to being on an airplane – looking at the passing views and the people sitting around. It's a time to stop and think.

Catching the tram is easy for me because the one I travel on is accessible. The accessible trams in Melbourne are wonderful. They were one of the main reasons why I decided to live in Melbourne after my MS was diagnosed. Trams were introduced into Melbourne in the 1930s and grew into an extensive network. But it's only been in recent years that changes have been made to some of the routes to make them more accessible for wheelchair users. Low-floor trams have been introduced and what the locals called 'super stops' have been built.

The super stops have platforms elevated up from the road with ramp access at one or both ends. The 109-tram route near where I live is one of those new accessible routes into the city.

The low-floor trams have entries level with the platforms. There's a special set of doors with wheelchair signs on them. That's where the 'bridging plate' is located – a metal plate running the width of one pair of tram doors that comes out from underneath to cover the gap between the tram and the platform. I have to alert the driver to activate it by waving a hand as the tram approached. I can also alert the driver to put the plate out for me before I get off. There's a blue wheelchair sign on a button inside the tram to press.

There are some trams where the bridging plate mechanism doesn't work. The gap between the tram floor and the platform can then be too wide for small wheels. There can also be a height difference from tram to tram and it isn't always level. If I think my scooter won't ride in, I have to get off and get help. Fortunately, Sue always comes with me.

The new low-floor trams are also air-conditioned. That's great when Melbourne gets hot with its 40°C temperatures.

Crowds are another consideration on the trams. I try to time my appointments or visits to be out of peak hours. Having no crowds makes it much easier. If it's crowded, Sue needs to help clear the way ahead for me.

Catching a tram for the first time on my scooter did feel a bit odd, but I became used to it and now, once on, I always sit back and enjoy being there. Tram-catching has become routine for me just as airports have. Only non-routine things stand out. The sound of the tram along the tramlines has a regularity and rhythm to it. It allows my mind to drift off into another land once I'm on board.

When I went by tram to see my GP in July, the closest super stop was at the very top of one of the busiest streets in Melbourne – Collins Street. It used to be Melbourne's only main street and has seen so much history happen in it since its construction in the early 1800s. It has always been busy, with a multitude of people walking hurriedly along the footpaths. John Brack tried to capture that busy scene in the 1950s with his painting *Collins St., 5 pm.*

I love John Brack's paintings and have been to a few exhibitions of his works. He preferred to paint people rather than landscapes. He once said that if someone could describe a painting in words there was no point in painting it. I like that, and I think words couldn't really describe the movement of people in his painting of Collins Street. There was much more in it than just a lot of people.

The top end of Collins Street where I get off the tram is known as the 'Paris' end because of its fine Victorian architecture and, in more recent times, because of its luxury stores, such as Giorgio Armani and Gucci. My GP's rooms are in an old, heritage-listed, seven-storey building built in the late 1920s.

There's a small step up from the footpath into the main entrance of the old building. It was too high for my scooter to go over so I had to get off. Sue lifted it over for me.

Once inside, I went into the small lift and up to the floor of the surgery. My doctor's waiting room is small so I parked my scooter just outside the glass doors. I said hello to the secretary, told her my name and took a seat in the waiting room.

Sue came with me and waited for me while I saw the doctor. I needed her for the tram gap, the crowd and the front step, as well as for help opening the waiting-room door. Most of all, I needed her for the security she gave me. I never liked the idea of going into the city on my own on any electric wheelchair or scooter. I wasn't confident enough. If something went wrong with the wheelchair or the battery, I wouldn't be able to manage on my own. When things have gone wrong before, Sue has always been there.

Once, a few years ago, I took my red indoor electric wheelchair into the city. As I was crossing the road, the wheels caught in the tramline in the middle of the road. The green 'walk' light soon changed to red. Engines were revving to come towards me. I couldn't move my chair. There was a big scramble with Sue and a few other people coming to help. For a moment, it was a bit scary.

Sue liked reading the recipes in the *Delicious* magazines in the doctor's waiting room. Sometimes she found one that she really wanted to keep. She'd say something to the secretary and there was an offer to photocopy it. It was an offer that was quickly accepted and the recipe would soon turn into dinner a night or so afterwards.

When it was my turn, the doctor came out and raised her arm for me. I held on to her with my left hand and walked with the walking stick down into her consultation room. 'How's your new scooter going? I saw it out there.'

'Really well. It's fantastic.'

'I've received all the reports about the melanoma on your toe. You should just need regular follow-up now. Is the dermatologist going to do that or the plastic surgeon?'

'The dermatologist.'

'And I can see you've been for a follow-up of your MS too. Good reports there on Tysabri. What can I do for you today?'

'I need some more Pravastatin and another letter for travelling to say what medications I'm on. Oh, and I'll need some scripts for a few things to take with me in case I need them.'

'Where are you off to this time?

'Norway and the Arctic.' I told her about the cruise.

'I think it's wonderful that you get out and about. I've told so many others about your new scooter. I hope it works out well for you on the overseas trip.'

'Thanks.'

She wrote out the prescriptions I needed and then wrote a letter for me to take travelling. This is what she wrote:

> ... is a patient of mine. She suffers from Secondary Progressive Multiple Sclerosis and is having infusions of Tysabri each 4 weeks with good effect. She has medications with her for her own personal use, including:
>
> Pravastatin
> Vitamin D
> Prednisolone

Maxolon
Imodium
Ibuprofen
Keflex

The Pravastatin was for my high cholesterol and the Vitamin D for my MS. The Prednisolone was in case I had an exacerbation of MS and needed to take a brief course. My neurologist said he'd be surprised if I needed it. But I took it in case.

The Maxolon was in case of nausea or vomiting and the Imodium in case I had diarrhoea. I'd never needed either of those, but I still took them travelling. The Ibuprofen was in case I strained a muscle. Keflex was in case I needed antibiotics.

We chatted for a little while about travelling and she checked my blood pressure. With my new prescriptions in hand and a new letter about my medications, I thanked her and left. Then Sue and I went down into the city to do some shopping before returning home on the tram.

Robin, an old friend, came over from the UK to stay on 3 August. I hadn't seen her for a few years. She was originally from Brisbane but had moved to London years ago to marry and settle there. The rest of her family followed over the years; even her mother moved over there when she was quite old. I thought it was fascinating that a whole family from Brisbane ended up moving to London to live.

A few days after Robin arrived, we saw on the evening news that there were riots, looting and arson attacks taking place in London. It was frightening. We followed the events in the news and Robin checked with family back home that they were all right. They were, but we still followed the news closely with her.

We weren't flying through London in September and we weren't staying there. But, somehow, something about it was unsettling. Perhaps it was because we were going to travel overseas soon. Perhaps I had to have another level of awareness when I was travelling about things going wrong or being in the wrong place at the wrong time. It seemed to be a new kind of behaviour too.

Robin had been to Melbourne before but that was a very long time ago. The top ten things for visitors to do in Melbourne include the Royal Botanic Gardens near Government House. We took Robin there, and then, the day after, also threw in a trip to the Royal Botanic Gardens, Cranbourne. The gardens at Cranbourne are set in native bushland about an hour-and-a-half's drive south-east of Melbourne. There's a stunning Australian Garden with native plants from every state and climate on display. One special feature is the Red Sand Garden, made to look and feel as if you are in the red centre of Australia.

Although another of the 'top things to see' was St Patrick's (Catholic) Cathedral, we instead went to St Paul's (Anglican) Cathedral on Flinders Street. An acquaintance in London had recommended that Robin see it. None of us had been inside before and we all thought it was great. I especially enjoyed the blue-coloured stone stripes in the sandstone pillars. They looked a bit Moorish and exotic.

We also drove Robin down the bayside to a pub in Portsea for lunch on the lawn. The lawn rolls down to Port Phillip Bay and looks back to the city of Melbourne. On the way home, Robin and Sue also did a walk out on the pier at St Kilda to see the penguins, near their rookeries on the rock break wall. It was good to be a tourist in our own town for a while. I practised using my new camera before I left on our trip.

Then we drove Robin to Canberra in Sue's still-feeling-new car. There was no more work done on the trip or bookings for the next few weeks.

The event in the news that was more relevant to our upcoming trip than the London riots happened on 5 August. That was the date of the Svalbard polar-bear attack. A group of schoolboys from Britain were camping in the Svalbard, somewhere on the island of Spitsbergen. A polar bear had wandered into the campsite at night and killed a boy. That was very sad news but we'd definitely not be camping in Spitsbergen.

The fallout from the global financial crisis of the previous years was also still reverberating. The stock market had reached another low point and share prices had fallen again. I'd been buying shares on and off at low prices. In between doing bookings, I'd check on the price of different stocks and see what was happening. In August, I bought some ANZ bank shares for AUD$19.57. I was pleased with myself for getting them at that price, but time would tell. I wasn't always successful with my purchases. Following the Australian share market was one of my interests and I enjoyed doing it.

Robin was in Canberra to go to the Australian Open Squash Championships and watch her daughter play, as well as catch up with family and friends. We stayed in Canberra too to watch some of the championships and check out a few art galleries. I saw Nicol David, the world number one women's squash champion, play. That was an amazing game; the difference between her and any other number was enormous. She was streets ahead of everyone.

Sue and I had both played squash when we were younger, after playing tennis years before. I played A Grade for Sydney University. Sue played State Grade and had been in the British Open Squash Championships. Playing squash was how Sue snapped a ligament in her knee. That was many years ago and they didn't repair those injuries then. She stopped playing squash and she still felt the effects of that injury in her knee. But it didn't stop her walking eighteen holes of golf!

I used to play squash with Carolyn too, at night, when I was living in Brisbane. After a few meetings and games, Carolyn had said, 'Let's do some training exercises instead of playing a game.' Playing a game with her was a waste of time. Carolyn was streets ahead of me.

We left Robin in Canberra to continue on her way. She was heading to Brisbane before she flew home. She was going to catch up with Carolyn, who she went to primary school with. They were still good friends.

Then we were back in Melbourne with two-and-a-half weeks to go before we left. It was time to look at the train timetables and the Nutshell trip again. I thought I'd try and finally do at least some of the bookings that I was sure of, instead of waiting to do them all at the same time.

I started with the first train trip leaving Bergen. But, on 15 August, when I tried to book the 8.40 a.m. train from Bergen to Myrdal for 22 September, it was unavailable! All bookings for it were blocked. I couldn't believe it.

With the planning before, I'd only been looking at the timetables. I'd never tried to actually make a booking. The first stage of doing the Nutshell links was no longer an option.

I had to think again and see what I could come up with to fit the kernel within the Nutshell into the trip.

CHAPTER 4

FINAL BOOKINGS AND PREPARATIONS

The shock stayed with me for a while. Why was nothing available? I wondered if that train from Bergen to Myrdal was unavailable because it was booked out. I knew our cruise ended in Bergen some days before and there'd be a lot of people disembarking. Surely there wouldn't be *that* many people, so many they'd take up a whole train, I thought. I should have booked it earlier. In my mind, and on paper, I'd lined up all the connecting times to flow from the train at 8.40 a.m. That would have to change.

When I looked again, it seemed as if repair work was taking place on some of the routes out of Bergen. The timetable had also changed by then and it looked quite different. There were segments between the connecting trains that had to be taken by bus. That would be yet another link to tackle! I didn't want that.

There was no 8.40 a.m. train from Bergen to Myrdal on 22 September. We wouldn't be able to make the ferry that I'd picked in Flåm. The next train to leave from Bergen that day was at 10.28 a.m., and it arrived at Myrdal at 12.20 p.m.

There was then a train leaving Myrdal at 1.27 p.m. that arrived in Flåm at 2.25 p.m. If we wanted to see the Nærøyfjord, we'd have to catch the last 3.10 p.m. ferry.

The 3.10 p.m. ferry was running at a very different schedule to the one I'd first chosen. It arrived in Gudvangen at 5.20 p.m. and didn't go back to Flåm on the same day. The option of going from and back to Flåm on the same ferry was gone. Once again – and the situation was even worse now – I wondered how would we'd get back. It was all happening much later in the day and left us less time.

I was in a slight panic. It was August and we were going early next month! I hadn't even booked us back to Oslo to catch the plane home yet!

At some stage, Carolyn suggested that we might decide not to go on the Nærøyfjord at all. We might just stay in Flåm, walk around and enjoy the place. There were a few things to see there. 'The waterway is right there in front of you and there are some walks,' she said. 'Then you could get the Flåm train back up again. At least you'd have been on the Flåm Line.' Mmm.

In the midst of this new flurry, the most amazing insight into the whole issue of the Nutshell happened. Carolyn had left me some maps of the Nutshell area, which showed various possible activities. She had collected them while she was there. I loved maps even more than I usually did after I looked at these ones. I saw a tunnel. The tunnel went through the mountain between Gudvangen and Flåm. There was a road in the tunnel and I wondered if a bus went that way.

I Googled 'bus timetable Gudvangen to Flåm' – and there it was. Yes, there was a public bus on that route! It didn't run often, only two or three times a day. There was one time on 22 September that fitted well with arriving by ferry from Flåm at 5.20 p.m. The bus left Gudvangen at 6.25 p.m. It seemed it wasn't the kind of bus for which you needed to pre-purchase a ticket. It was all looking good.

I was so excited about finding that tunnel. It looked like it was only twenty minutes between Gudvangen and Flåm. It was a public bus service. They'd have to take my scooter, I thought. But where was the bus stop? It couldn't be that far away. We'd work that out later. I'd ask a few more questions when we were in Norway.

Finally, I had another Nutshell side trip organised, with a set of transport links that fitted well together and were even better than my original plans. It was okay to have waited.

I felt confident and went ahead with booking the train journey parts with NSB. I started at the end of the trip, getting us back to Oslo first, a trip that began at Flåm the day after we'd done the Nutshell. The bookings were for 23 September on the 11 a.m. Flåm Line train leaving Flåm, and then the 12.25 p.m. train leaving Myrdal for Oslo. Those train times hadn't changed and were still available.

I then went ahead with the train bookings from Bergen, starting at 10.28 a.m., for the day before. And then all the NSB bookings were done.

I called out to Sue who was watering the balcony garden. 'I've finished!' I don't think she heard me. So I told her again later.

With those bookings done, it was just a matter of doing all the usual last minute things, such as having my Tysabri infusion, getting a haircut and doing the packing.

My thirty-third infusion was on 17 August; it was a Wednesday, a day that fitted in well with Sue's golf. And it was easy to remember the same day of the week each time. Having an infusion was just another routine for me.

We left home at the usual time to go to the hospital, about 10.20 a.m. I went through the door of our apartment on my walker, with the freshly charged battery on its seat, to catch the lift down to the car park. Sue's car space was right beside the lifts. I got out of the lift, walked only a few metres to park my walker and left it at the end of the car space. Then I got into the car with the help of my walking stick and Sue's arm.

Sue put the battery in the car and then collected my collapsed scooter from the storage area nearby. She wheeled it to the back of the car to put it into the boot. The scooter was in good working order again. The broken locking clips had been replaced, and Jetstar had reimbursed the full cost. It had also been checked and freshened up ready for travel.

The drive to the hospital took only about ten to fifteen minutes. My appointment in the Day Surgery/Day Oncology Centre was at 11.00 a.m. That was the usual time. I'd booked the dates and that time about six to twelve months ahead.

We drove along Royal Parade looking for a parking spot. We found a free space in a two-hour ticketed parking zone, a few streets away from the hospital. All the disabled parking areas were usually full by that time. After we parked the car, I put my disabled person's parking permit on the dashboard near the car registration sticker in the windscreen. That would give us four hours free parking, double the usual time and with no ticket to pay for. That disabled parking permit was a fantastic thing to have.

I got out and used the rails on the top of the car to help me walk down along the top of the gutter to the boot. Sometimes it felt as though I had ten-kilogram weights attached to my legs. They'd feel so heavy and I moved so slowly.

Sue got the scooter out, rolled it off the road and up over the gutter on to the verge. Then she put the seat up, lifted the steering tiller up, checked the battery connection and unlocked the wheels. The power light flashed red and it was ready to go. I stepped out, got on and rode the scooter across the grass on to the footpath. I waited for Sue.

We went along footpaths in front of the fine old Victorian buildings lining Royal Parade. Some of them had signs out the front indicating they were part of the University of Melbourne's Conservatorium of Music. One indicated that it was an 'Early Music Studio'. Another old building had a large sign that said 'Trinity College and the University of Melbourne', with arrows showing the direction to 'English for Academic Purposes'. Some buildings looked like private houses, with gardens that had been established many decades ago out the front. When the gardens were in flower, they looked beautiful. It was the last month of winter by then and the camellias were still in flower, along with some snowbells.

'That's *Camellia sasanqua*, I think' said Sue. Then I thought she said, 'Or is it *meticularis*?'

'*Meticularis*?' I repeated. That last one sounded like me, I thought.

'No, *reticulata*! Anyway, I think it's a *sasanqua*.'

'Okay.' I hadn't heard properly. But I still thought to myself that it was a bit of a funny mistake – *meticularis*!

It was about 13°C and I had my scarf firmly around my neck. I put my head down against the wind as I scooted down the footpaths. No time for looking at more flowers. We crossed about three roads to get to the hospital entrance.

As I went over the last crossroad, the one just before the University High School, the scooter stopped. It happened after going over the bump of the rise from road to footpath. I was still learning how high I could go, but I'd made it over that bump many times before. Fortunately, the car approaching on my right stopped. I got off, grabbed my half-folded walking stick lying on the base of the scooter and unlocked the wheels. Sue soon caught up with me (this scooter went a little faster than Sue could walk, and Sue was a fast walker). We rolled the scooter up over the rise and on to the footpath. 'What happened?' asked Sue.

'I think the battery jumped out. It just stopped after the bump. The light's gone off too.'

'You should take it at an angle.'

'Maybe the battery isn't in firmly enough,' I answered.

Sue took out the battery and fitted it back in again, pulling the Velcro ties firmly over each other. She checked the light. Yes, it was on and the scooter was working again.

Well, I thought, I really must keep that in mind when I'm out on the scooter in the future. Make sure the battery is in firmly and try not to go over too high a bump or a rise. Take it at an angle when safe, or stop, get out and move the scooter manually.

As I was swiftly moving along again, an older man in a suit saw me and called out, 'Oh, I like your Ferrari!' He was smiling and giving big nods of approval.

I smiled back and said, 'Thanks, but it's a Lamborghini!' He laughed loudly. My scooter was yellow, not red.

We didn't lose too much time with all the goings-on along the way, only a few minutes. We went a bit further along the footpath and then turned right to go around the back of Melbourne Private Hospital. I went along the footpath beside the road into the Royal

Melbourne Hospital car park. The sign, high up on a post at the corner of Royal Parade, read 'Car Park Full'. It usually said that. There was another large red sign just before a boom gate in front of the car park. It read, 'Sorry, Car Park Near Capacity, Card Holders Only'. That sign always seemed to be there too.

Around the next corner and to my right was a very modern, tall building. It had a large sign at the top saying, 'Walter + Eliza Hall'; it was the medical research institute. I turned left, went down the ramp and through the automatic doors into the private hospital's main entry area. That was where the booking area and the lifts were. The Day Centre was only twenty metres along on the right on the ground floor. I didn't need to take the lift.

'Hello, Gracie,' I said when I reached the small reception desk.

'Hello, Maureen. How are you?'

'I'm well, thanks. How are you?'

'I'm fine,' she said. 'Any change of address to report? Are these details still correct?' She showed me the sticker on my admission form. It was the Informed Financial Consent form noting my private health insurance and status for payment.

'No changes, all correct', I said, after looking. I signed the form.

'Have you been overseas in the last two weeks?' This was followed by the familiar question, 'To the best of your knowledge, have you been in contact with anyone with the SARS virus or do you have any SARS symptoms?' This was the routine now before proceeding to the next step of admission. The concern about the spread of SARS (Severe Acute Respiratory Syndrome) came from the experience of swine flu, and the knowledge that an infectious, life-threatening respiratory illness could follow. The hospital was trying to take precautions.

'No to all of those. But, Grace, I *am* going away soon,' I said excitedly.

Grace filled out the form by ticking my answers and said, 'Oh, great, where are you going this time?'

'Norway, the Arctic and North Pole areas. There's a cruise,' I answered.

'Oh, good, sounds interesting. Take this form with you through to the chairs. I think they're ready for you.'

Sue went ahead to check. The day surgery patients were in beds in the area to my left and the adapted former two-bed hospital space used for day chemotherapy was further in and to the right. I rode my scooter down into that area. There were four large recliner chairs spread out in the room. Three chairs were on one side and one was on the other, next to a low desk. Two nurses were busy with the other patients, but Jen looked up and said, 'Hi, Maureen, you can take that chair over there in the corner,' nodding her head in its direction.

It wasn't the flashest-looking private hospital day centre that I'd ever been in. But all the nurses there were good, the chairs were comfortable and that's where they delivered the Tysabri for patients with private health insurance.

I liked the chair that Jen had nodded to. It was near a frosted window, from which the sun came in, and against a wall. I put my walking stick in the corner after Sue helped me over. It was warm in that spot and no one would try to get past me. I got into the chair and started to work the electronic controls. I adjusted the back and the lower leg sections of the reclining chair so I could stretch my legs out and up a little. Meantime, Sue rode off on the scooter to park it in the waiting area. But before Sue left, Jen looked up from writing some notes. She said to Sue, 'So, where are you going shopping today? DJs or Myers?'

Sue laughed and said, 'Yes, I read that there're some specials on.' She added, 'Do you have any more new handbags yet?'

Jen laughed too, saying, 'I wish! See you later.'

I got my book and my glasses out, and put them on the wide arm ledge that folded out. I put my left arm on a pillow. The nurse who was helping Jen that day came over and said, 'Hi, I'm Ami. I'll just do your obs.' She proceeded to put a blood pressure cuff on my arm and then pressed a button on a small machine on wheels. It recorded my blood pressure, which read 130 on 75. Ami wrote the numbers down. Next, she placed a plastic clip on my finger. It had a lead attached to the same machine. By 'O2', the machine read '99'. Then Ami placed a temperature probe with a fresh earpiece in my ear and clicked it. Ami said, '36.8°C. Normal.' Then she gave me a form.

The form was a pre-infusion questionnaire. I completed one every time I received my infusion of Tysabri. There were seven statements on the form with boxes beside them. Above the column of boxes were the words, 'Please initial the boxes.' Examples of the seven statements are:

> Prior to this infusion, I have discussed with my neurologist any new or worsening medical problems (such as new or sudden changes in my thinking, eyesight, balance, strength or other problems) that lasted or worsened over several days.
> I have asked my caregiver and they have not noticed any differences in my personality, thinking abilities or behaviour.
> I have a copy of the Consumer Medicine Information (CMI) and Patient Alert Card for Tysabri. I have read the CMI within the last 24 hours.

I had to read the statements on the form, initial the boxes, sign and date it before handing it back to the nurse.

The statement about differences in personality or behaviour was an interesting one. I'd ask Sue as she drove me to my infusion. She'd often say, 'No worse than usual!' On that day, I think Sue had said, 'Nothing that you can't make up for.' Mmm, I thought. It was her birthday in a few days. Of course, I knew she really meant she hadn't noticed any differences and I could initial that box.

The one about reading the CMI I interpreted as being about possible litigation on my part. My neurologist had given me a CMI booklet to read before receiving Tysabri. I initialled that box.

I initialled the rest of the boxes, signed the form and handed it back to Ami. 'Thanks.'

A few minutes later, Jen came over to the trolley sitting against the far wall. She used the hand sanitiser sitting above it on the wall. Jen then made up the Tysabri pack. The Tysabri was in a small plastic bag with my name on it. The pharmacy had delivered it not long before. She added some 0.9% normal saline to the contents of the Tysabri bag with a sterile needle. She hooked the little bag on to the drip stand. It joined a 500-millilietre plastic bag of 0.9% normal saline that was already hanging there. Jen connected the tubing coming out of the two bags to each other. She turned off the Tysabri and flushed the saline through the long tubing that ended on the pillow where my arm was lying. All the air was now out of the tubing and Jen turned the flow off.

It was time for the needle. Most of the time, the needle went in on the first go. It'd only been about three times that it hadn't. I had good, juicy veins that stood out. It shouldn't be difficult. The Tysabri didn't seem to damage my veins either. The needles looked a bit like the old scalp vein needles, but they were more modern ones with a long needle. They had to be pulled back a little before advancing. Once, when the needle didn't seem to go in at first, it was because the nurse was new and not familiar with the technique. Jen never missed; she was an old hand. The tiniest pinch of pain was all I usually felt.

Once everything was flowing and the saline had gone into me, Jen stopped it and turned the Tysabri on. She placed the drip tubing inside an infusion pump mounted on the intravenous drip stand. The metal drip stand itself was on five wheels and moved freely to be right beside me. Jen set the counting device. She pressed the buttons to get the machine to deliver the entire contents of the little bag over a period of one hour.

I sat back and looked around. There was no one there whom I recognised that day. The other three patients were all older men. I think they had either bladder cancer or prostate cancer. Their chemotherapy was running and they all looked okay. There weren't usually any other people at the centre receiving Tysabri when I was there.

I was reading Anna Funder's new book *All That I Am*. I was really enjoying it. It's great that she's an Australian writer, and that she'd grown up in Melbourne.

Two of the patients were chatting to each other and one was reading the *Herald Sun*. I put my head down and got stuck into my book.

After an hour, at about 12.10 p.m., the beep, beep of the drip counter alarm went off. Jen came over and flushed through the remaining Tysabri in the line with the saline. 'We have to get all the good stuff in,' she said. Then she said, 'I'm going to Africa soon. I can't wait. I need a holiday.'

'Wow,' I said. 'That's fantastic. Tell me exactly where you're going.' I hadn't been to Africa but I thought about it every now and then. Jen told me about a cheap tour she'd found. She was going with a friend whom she hadn't travelled with before so she was a little apprehensive. She already knew I was going to Norway and the nearby icy-cold areas. She, on the other hand, liked hot and sunny spots.

The saline flowed for another hour through the drip counter machine. I didn't feel any different after the infusion or in the time leading up to it. I had never had a reaction to Tysabri and I didn't that time either.

It was supposed to be the long-term benefits that counted. I did feel better with all the infusions I'd had so far. I had more energy and was able to walk a bit more often. It seemed like my MS had stopped progressing too. I was very happy on Tysabri, unlike some earlier treatments I'd had.

I was glad I'd stopped those earlier injections. I gave them to myself three times a week. They made me feel worse. After a few years, I discussed the situation with my neurologist. I didn't know if I was feeling awful because of the injections or because of my MS. I thought that if I stopped the injections, I'd know what I was dealing with.

So I stopped them. I felt better but my MS did progress. Then along came Tysabri. With all its risks, I still thought it was worthwhile trying. I was so pleased that I did.

Having my infusions always followed the same routine. It was just part of my life. Again, I'd only really notice things if they were different, such as the time the nurse ran the saline first for an hour instead of the Tysabri and none of us noticed! Most other times, all went well and there was nothing in particular to note.

The most enjoyable part of the trip was the coffee at a cafe afterwards. The day centre was in a great area of Melbourne, where a lot was going on. I used my 2010 edition of the *Melbourne Coffee Review: A Guide to Melbourne's Top 100 Coffee Spots* to find a different place every time. I wanted to experience as many as possible. I turned the book into a bit of a diary, adding new cafes as I discovered them. I wrote an article for *DiVine* in July 2011 about good coffee and the cafes that were the most accessible. I was going to write another piece and give the cafes a star or bean rating, using both coffee quality and accessibility together. The timing of the infusions fitted in perfectly with lunch and coffee afterwards.

That day we went to Pope Joan, a cafe in Brunswick, not far away. Pope Joan wasn't in my guidebook but I'd read a review of it in *The Age's* Tuesday Epicure section. I was testing it out.

I really like the name Pope Joan. The story that goes with the name is interesting too. Many hundreds of years ago, there was supposed to have been a female pope, who disguised herself as a man. Her disguise fell apart when, during a big ceremonial street procession, she went into labour and delivered a baby in the street. Amazing!

The cafe had great food, great coffee and it was sort of accessible. The entry ramp was at an odd angle and wasn't easy.

On the way home, we stopped at South Melbourne Markets. That was also the usual routine. But time was counting down now for our trip away and we didn't need much fresh food. Sue bought just a few things.

When I arrived home and checked the phone, there was a message from Mum. 'Oh, it's just Mum here, love … nothing urgent. It's, ah, about a quarter to four and, ah, I'll give you a ring a little bit later. You might be out or, ah, I'm not sure if you're having your immusions today, ah, or not, but, ah, I'll give you a ring, nothing urgent. I'll give you a ring back in about half an hour, love. Okay, lovey. Thank you very much, love. Uum, umm, it's Wednesday. Thank you.'

Mum's messages seemed to be getting longer and longer as she got older. She also seemed to be thanking people more often. We talked to each other at least two or three times a week. She'd update me on what was happening in her life and check how I was going. I was at home when she rang again. 'How did you go with your fusion, love?' She had a bit of trouble with the word 'infusion'. Once she called it my 'emersion'!

'Fine, thanks, Mum. How are you?' Sometimes she'd take forty-five minutes without a break to answer that question! All was fine with her, too. There was nothing wrong. I didn't want her to become more unwell before I left or while I was away. She was trying some new pills for her back that seemed to be helping. So that was great.

Mum was the only person in the world who could call me 'love' and I wouldn't take umbrage. Sue wasn't offended either. It was possibly because Mum would also use our names and she'd called me 'love' and other nicknames ever since I could remember.

Most of my friends didn't like being called 'love' or 'dear'. Sue could get particularly upset when it was people who were providing a service. She'd reply, 'That's so disappointing, you calling me that. It's so unprofessional.' My friend Jan in Tasmania would say, 'Don't call me "pet"!' while others might respond, 'Don't "darl" me, I'm not your darl.' But Mum used 'love' and she said it with love.

Sue had one special golf competition to take part in before we left for our trip. It was a team event called 'Elizabethan foursomes'. That sounded like a dance to me, but, of course, it wasn't. Sue would be away for most of the daylight hours, what with all that was involved in this event.

Long before I woke, on that special day, Sue had left. I got up and went to the kitchen. As expected, Sue had left my cereal bowl on the bench, filled with her homemade muesli mix and covered with Gladwrap. An orange, half a pear and a Lady Finger banana were beside it on a cutting board. All I had to do was stand at the kitchen bench, take the peeled orange out of the Gladwrap and cut up the other fruit to go on the muesli. The fridge was immediately behind me and it was easy to turn around to face it. I could get the natural yoghurt and the skim milk out of the fridge to go on top of the muesli.

There was a note beside the fruit with a list of foods to remind me of what Sue had organised for lunch, in case I couldn't wait for her to come home late in the afternoon. It read:

> Salmon in bowl (RHS)
> Carrot (use ones in left drawer)
> Mushroom
> Leaves in server (already washed)
> Cucumber (R drawer)
> Toms (top of dresser)
> Bread in freezer
> Apple (use left front)

I could do some food preparation but Sue was in charge of all food arrangements. I was slow and my left hand was not the same as it used to be.

***

The problem with my left hand is that it's weak and doesn't move smoothly. When I make rapid alternating movements, my hand becomes jerky and slow, and loses its normal smoothness. This symptom is called dysdiadochokinesia. When this symptom is present, it means there's something wrong with a part of the brain.

I was taught the name, the meaning and the relevance of this symptom when I was a medical student, and I tested patients for it when I was in clinical practice as a doctor. I'd ask them to do a pointing test. They'd point at something with their right forefinger and then do it again with their left one. In recent times, since I've become a patient myself, my neurologist tests me for dysdiadochokinesia each time he performs his routine neurological examination.

Chopping vegetables is a little difficult. Not that I've ever chopped vegetables in any rapid, skilled way like my brother, who taught commercial cooking at TAFE, or like a chef on television. My hand movements just became clumsier than they used to be, making it harder to prepare meals. I can't stand up in one place for very long either.

It also became harder to carry plates. I can't walk and carry a plate at the same time any more. My two hands are occupied in trying to help me balance when I move. For carrying plates, I often put them on the seat of my walker to move them from one place to another. It isn't a bad serving-trolley but it's limited in the number of plates it can carry.

When we have friends over to dinner, I sometimes feel funny that I can't help serve courses while people are sitting at the dining table. Clearing plates away isn't easy either. But most times everybody jumps in and helps, and Sue doesn't need my help at all.

I used to get annoyed with myself for not being able to do such simple things properly. But, as time has passed, and as Sue has been so good about taking on all the food-related aspects of living and doing them so well, I've become completely accepting. I know I do other things that come more easily to me, that also contribute to our living arrangements. This makes acceptance easier.

The kitchen bench works well for moving plates. It's long and extends down from in front of the fridge to the small square dining table near the window. After I've put my breakfast or lunch on to a plate, I slide it down from one end to another, or lift it up and down in little steps along the bench. Then I can lift it off at the end and put it on the table.

The most important spots on the bench top are the corners at the ends. I always make sure those ends are free, with nothing on top, so they're ready to grab and hold as I move past.

Sometimes, as I slide a plate down the bench top, it might quickly flash through my mind that I'm doing all this because I can't carry a plate and walk at the same time any more. I don't ever dwell on it. It's just a flash, a thought brushing past. I quickly and happily let my mind drift off to the sound of the music coming from ABC Classic FM on the radio. Then I sit down to eat and read.

***

I finished preparing breakfast and enjoyed it while reading *The Age*. After breakfast, I wanted to have one more look at the Nutshell trip.

All the train bookings were finished. It was just those two bookings in the middle that were left – the ferry and the bus on 22 September.

There was another website for the Fjord1 ferry, with a timetable. Along with the times, there was a warning that by that time of year, the service was weather-dependent, and it would close fully at the end of September. I assumed that was because it would be winter, with snow and ice about. I also assumed the word '*Kai*', which appeared after 'Flåm' and 'Gudvangen' on the timetable, meant 'quay' or 'pier' and the times listed were when the ferry would be at those places. The website allowed me to book ahead of time and pay online.

By that time, I thought I'd done enough and would wait until we were in Norway to do that booking. From the emails going back and forth with the local tourist office, I felt that the ferry trip would not be booked up. There were no specific seats allocated when you bought tickets anyway. From Carolyn's photos of the ferry and from the website photos, it looked like everyone just piled on.

I didn't look at the bus timetable again. I thought I'd worried enough and that we'd just work it out when we got there. I stopped thinking about it and began to prepare to leave.

When Sue came home and I asked how she went, she said, 'We all played well and tried our best, but we were runners-up.' She was carrying a box. 'There's a nice set of wine glasses in here, and they're both engraved. Look.' Sue proudly opened the box and showed me.

'Congratulations! Well done. What a nice prize.'

Prizes won and bookings done, it was soon time for a haircut.

I went down to the car with Sue, using my walker, and got into the passenger seat. I used my walker to help me get to the hairdresser, not my scooter. Sue took the walker, flipped the seat up, brought the legs and wheels together and then put it sideways on the back seat. She drove me to my hairdresser in Port Melbourne for a 4.30 p.m. appointment.

When we reached Bay Street, Sue was able to park the car nearby, about ten to fifteen metres away from the front door of a salon called Silky Waves. That was great; it was only a short walk for me. After Sue got the walker out and brought it around for me to use, she said, 'Anything we need at Coles that you can think of?'

'Oh, maybe some more skim milk. And the toilet paper is a bit low. I think that's all.' Sue usually did some supermarket shopping for the forty or so minutes that I was at the hairdresser.

'Hello, my lady,' Dimitrios greeted me as he rushed to open the front door of his salon. He helped me get the walker up the little step from the footpath into the salon. Lisa, his wife, was there and she greeted me too. She was also a hairdresser but she mainly ran the beauty side of their business while Dimitrios did most of the hairdressing. He was born in Greece. 'Do you have another trip planned yet?' he asked as I sat down.

'I haven't been on this trip yet,' I replied. 'We leave this Thursday.'

'Oh, yes, you said you were going somewhere in Norway, didn't you? I look forward to seeing your photos when you get back. You must remember to send them to me. By Picasa, wasn't it? My email address is the same. I have saved the Egypt ones in a special place.'

'Yes, sure.'

I enjoyed talking with Dimitrios and listening to what he had to say about Greek culture, customs and habits. He and Lisa's family were from the island of Lesvos. They were married there in 2002 and moved to Australia in 2004. In 2005, they bought the hairdressing business in Bay Street and have been there ever since.

I told Dimitrios that, many years ago, I'd been to his island in Greece. I thought it was sometime in the early 1990s, on the way home after a conference in Edinburgh. I'd spent about a week there.

While there, I went on a one-day trip to Turkey and back. The ferry left from the island's capital of Mytilini and in about an hour it was in Ayvalik, Turkey. It was a very interesting day trip, especially the drive to Pergamum to see the Roman ruins.

'Is it a long one or short one today, Maureen?' asked Dimitrios.

'It's been a bit over five weeks this time. I think I need a short one.'

Sometimes I just had a trim. I thought Dimitrios was a good hairdresser. He'd done his training in Greece and had a long family history in hairdressing. I'm sure I always looked much better when I left!

After about forty minutes, I met up with Sue, who was waiting outside in the car.

Back home, we just had to finish the packing and we'd be ready to go. We'd been putting clothes out in a designated area for the last week and it was down to the final steps now. 'What else needs washing?' I asked Sue. 'Let's look at the list again.'

A little later on, when we were watching the seven o'clock ABC News, Sue said, 'Look at what those people are wearing.' The footage was in Oslo.

There was still a lot of information being broadcast about the Norway bombing and the massacre that had occurred the month before, in late July. Flowers were being left at the cathedral near the government offices that had been bombed. It was a terrible series of events, and seventy-seven people had died. Newspaper articles said that it was 'the worst peacetime massacre in the country'. Norway was supposed to be such a peaceful country, the home of the Nobel Peace Prize.

The people on the news were wearing very warm clothes, but it was supposed to be summer there. 'Let's just check we have enough warm clothes,' said Sue. 'You know, we mustn't pack too much, though. We have to travel light. We always seem to take things that we don't need.'

'I don't think we can get much lighter than seventeen kilograms for one bag,' I replied. 'And I always make a list so we can look back at it for help next time. I really think we should be packing things in the bag right now.'

We spent the next few days packing on and off.

Sue rolled the clothes and packed them in an organised way into one medium-sized luggage bag. I sat on the bed and did a lot of clothes-rolling too.

Socks and other suitable items went inside shoes. For some things, we applied the rule 'one on, one off and one in the wash', taking three. We weren't going anywhere where we had to dress up. Smart casual was our highest dress code. None of our travel clothes needed ironing, just good rolling. We'd wear the heaviest shoes on the plane.

'What about the psyllium?' I asked.

'Oh yes, I suppose we should take our own in case we can't buy any when we get there.'

I've been putting psyllium on my breakfast cereal for years. I know the risk of bowel problems is high with MS. I try hard to make sure my diet is extra healthy. I try to drink enough water and have a lot of fresh fruit and vegetables. Psyllium adds some extra fibre. And 'oomph', I thought.

After we tucked the psyllium into a space in the luggage bag, it was on to packing the backpack. The Luggie scooter charger and other chargers for phones and cameras went in first. I didn't want to chance having any of those things lost along the way. I also packed my pills, the letters from my doctor and other important paperwork, such as the e-tickets, the hotel bookings and the like.

The backpack also had to take my new superzoom camera in its protective bag and Sue's video camera in its little makeshift case. The backpack was packed tightly and weighed just below seven kilograms.

As we packed, I made a list of the things we were taking to Norway. I had a basic packing list and always modified it for whatever trip was coming up. My packing list for Norway and the Arctic appears in Appendix 1.

I saved all the booking confirmations and most other documents into files on my computer and copied them on to a USB memory stick. I put the memory stick into a small travel wallet that I would wear on a belt around my waist.

The local currency in Norway was the Norwegian krone. I'd ordered some kroner about two weeks before and had already picked them up in South Yarra. There was a collocated Westpac Bank branch and American Express money exchange office there. It was very handy to be able to withdraw cash from one teller and immediately hand it over to the money exchange clerk. The cash notes in Norwegian kroner, equivalent to about AUD$1,000, went into my money belt.

Sue spoke with Ian, our apartment's resident manager, a few days before we left and asked if he would please collect our mail for us while we were away.

'Just leave me a note with the dates written on it in the little box outside the office.' Ian was terrific. I knew he would look after things.

I emailed copies of my travel table (Appendix 2) showing where we'd be on any given day to a few friends and family. I posted a paper copy to Mum. She liked to follow along and see where I was. One paper copy went into my documents pack. I wanted to take it with me to refer to and, when I got back, I could add in a 'final costs' column.

I also filled out the online form on the Australian Government Smart Traveller website to record where we'd be. Names of hotels, the cruise and contact numbers all went in just in case there was an emergency of any sort.

The big day finally came – 1 September. We had our bags packed, zipped up and ready. Sue brought some of the plants on the balcony inside to keep them somewhat watered while we were away. Alan's taxi arrived a little ahead of time and drove us to Melbourne (Tullamarine) International Airport.

Everything at the airport flowed smoothly, following the usual steps. Thai Airways allowed me to ride my scooter to the boarding gate. That was always the easiest way because then Sue didn't have to push me in a wheelchair with the backpack on her back, juggling the few other odds and ends that always seemed to appear as well.

When we were at the boarding gate, Thai Airways staff said I could ride my scooter along the air bridge to the aircraft entry door. Wow, that didn't happen very often! We boarded first and when I reached the plane door, I got off my scooter and helped Sue. I only helped with the first few steps of collapsing it down. Sue did the rest. Airport staff took the scooter and we boarded the plane.

We left Melbourne at 3 p.m. and we were soon safely up in the air. All the planning and important bookings were done. All the steps involved in getting to seat 41K were done. It was time to switch off and relax. There was that special feeling of being up in the air again. There were no loud sounds, just a low, hypnotic hum.

We stopped at Bangkok to change planes. When I was leaving the plane to get into the wheelchair that was waiting at the aircraft door, one of the Thai Airport workers greeted me with my scooter beside him. 'We thought you might want to use this. Do you want it? Or shall I take it with the baggage to be loaded?'

That was something else that hardly ever happened. I had to think quickly. We were going to change planes and go to another gate. It would be much better if an airport staff member wheeled me (with Sue close behind) to where we had to be. 'No, thank you, I won't use it. I'll be fine in the wheelchair. But thank you very much for bringing it up to me.'

We went to the next flight's boarding gate and waited a short time. Around midnight, we boarded the plane to Oslo and were soon in the air again. Mmmm, it was time to sleep.

PART THREE:
TRAVELLING

CHAPTER 1

OSLO

We arrived in Oslo on a beautiful sunny day. We were in Norway at last at 7.30 a.m. on Friday 2 September. All that planning, booking and preparing was in the past.

Our arrival at the airport was easy. We were off last as usual and there was a wheelchair waiting for me at the aircraft door. An attendant took us along the air bridge and then through to the baggage collection area. We picked up our one bag from the carousel and my yellow scooter from the fragile-luggage area. They'd both arrived without any problems. The scooter wasn't upside down on the moving carousel and we didn't have to go searching for it. We assembled it and it worked. All was in order.

One surprise, however, was that there was no customs check, or none that I noticed. Sue walked and I scootered straight out into the arrivals area. Then there, to our right in the distance, was the entrance to the fast train into the city, just as Carolyn had said. How easy, I thought, and also, why can't Melbourne Airport have something like this?

We collected a few brochures and asked questions at the tourist information desk before going to the train. I thought we'd be catching the train to Oslo Central Station to get to our accommodation.

'Where are you staying?' asked the helpful woman at the desk.

'The Frogner House Apartments, at Arbinsgate 3,' I replied.

'You can catch the train to the Nationaltheatret stop,' she said. 'Just stay on the train for two more stops after Oslo *sentralstasjon*. It will be just a short walk from there.' She showed me the route on an Oslo transport map. I looked at the map closely and the woman pointed the places out to us.

Straight away, I knew I had to change spellings and pronunciation in my mind. Yes, I was in a foreign country! I wanted to try and connect with the place as soon as I could, and recognise and try to use Norwegian words.

I quickly learned that Oslo Central Station was 'Oslo S' or 'Oslo *sentralstasjon*'. I'm not naturally good at learning languages. In fact, I'm hopeless at it, but I thought *sentralstasjon* wasn't too difficult even for me to remember!

We headed down towards the train, where we found that buying the tickets wasn't difficult either. There were several ticket-dispensing machines, all very visible, and they took credit cards. Two assistants came over quickly. 'Can we help you?'

'Thanks, but it looks like I just have to put my credit card in here and pick the stop.'

'Yes, that is all.'

Everyone at the airport was keen to offer assistance and they all spoke English well.

We took the lift to a platform that was one level below the arrival area. We showed our tickets as we went through the turnstile on to the platform. The platform signs in Norwegian took us a little while to figure out. The first train that arrived was going in the opposite direction to where we wanted to go; someone who was waiting there too, thoughtfully pointed this out to us.

Once the correct train arrived, boarding was only slightly difficult. After a flat entry, there were two steps up to get to the seats in the carriage. I climbed up and Sue dragged the bag and then the scooter up the steps and into the carriage.

The train to and from the airport was called the Flytoget fast train. It was modern, clean and had what seemed like mostly business people travelling to work. It took about fifty minutes to get to the city and, when we arrived at Nationaltheatret, it was still early in the morning, about 8.30 a.m.

I rang the Frogner House Apartments reservations desk as soon as we were up out of the underground platform and in the open air. They told me how to get to them to pick up the keys. We knew that we couldn't get into our apartment until after 3 p.m. But, in an earlier email, they'd said they'd try to let us in sooner if they could. It all depended on what was happening that morning.

Fredrik was at reception when we arrived – he was the person I'd emailed. The apartment was not quite ready. But we could leave our luggage with him and go off exploring while we waited.

The Frogner House business had three different groups of apartments in Oslo available for short-term bookings. The main reception desk for all of them was located in one set of apartments that were undergoing renovations. Fredrik showed us around its ground floor.

'We are including lifts in our new building work,' he said, pointing proudly to a small lift beside a grand old staircase. 'All the work here should be finished next January.'

'That's wonderful. You've thought about people who can't get up stairs easily or who need wheelchairs and other aids.'

'Yes, and we have thought about the bathrooms too. Our other buildings are very old. This is the first building for us to renovate.'

This place was several hundred metres away from the place we'd booked. By the time we reached Fredrik, the battery charge on my yellow scooter was close to zero. I carried the charging unit in a pack that sat over the back of the scooter seat – a scooter backpack. Fredrik helped us set up the scooter for charging over in a corner of the reception area.

The lithium battery in my yellow scooter lasted three to four hours if I used it continuously. If not used continuously, it would usually last all day. When I travelled, I was usually in continuous mode. I'd been using my scooter without charging it since we left the apartment in Melbourne.

Nearby, only about ten metres away on the street corner, was a wonderful-looking cafe. The coffee smelt good as we passed by and from the look of their machines it seemed like they served real coffee. Perfect, I thought. We'll leave the scooter charging and our bags at Frogner reception and go to the cafe. I walked there using my stick and holding Sue's arm.

At the cafe, we sat, looked around and just really enjoyed being in what felt like a wonderful, small, friendly city. We were in the diplomatic district of Oslo, the capital of Norway. It was the country's biggest city, with a population of about 600,000.

The coffee was good. We had a second cup. It tasted like a flat white but on the menu board it had a long Norwegian name beginning with 'L'. But it didn't look anything like the word 'latte'. Some people were having coffee out of what looked like soup bowls. Sue chatted to the barista to learn something about the coffee in Oslo. We soon learned that Norwegians were serious about their coffee, which was great news. The coffee in this cafe was just as good as some of the best I've had in Melbourne.

We also had a small baguette with *jamon* as a snack. I'm not sure what meal we were up to by then. It had been about thirty hours since we left home. It felt so good just being there, having coffee, sitting in the cafe, surrounded by both old and young people reading newspapers or chatting. It felt as if we'd been there for ages.

I'd heard of some famous names and places associated with Oslo. There was the Nobel Peace Centre, the Munch Museum, Vigeland Park, the *Kon-Tiki* raft and the ski jump for a start. That first day though, we thought we'd just wander around and try to get a feel for the place.

Feeling refreshed and invigorated after the coffee stop, we went back to collect the scooter. But before going out, I had to have my new camera. Sue got it out of the backpack for me. I always have a camera with me when I travel. Most of my photos have been taken while I was travelling. It's an important part of me and I have to have my camera close to hand all the time, ready to use.

I don't just point and shoot. I think about and feel a scene before I take the photo. Sometimes I appreciate and feel things more when I'm looking through a camera lens. And when I look at the photos later, I can connect with those feelings and become lost in the flood of memories that pour out of them. I can gaze at a photo for a long time, thinking and remembering.

The first photo I took in Oslo was of the coffee shop on the corner. The coffee and that wonderful feeling of being there are in that photo. It certainly won't win a competition, but, for me, the feeling and the memory are in it.

We then retraced some of our earlier steps, but we moved more slowly and with much more awareness of what was around us because we weren't going anywhere in particular.

I noticed a nice big park on the way from the Nationaltheatret stop, so we went back there. We went past the Nobel Institute with its cast bronze bust of Alfred Nobel on the front lawn. We stopped to look. This was the building where the Nobel Committee voted for the person who would win the peace prize. There was a new peace centre, open to the public, elsewhere, down at the waterfront. That was on our list for later.

When we reached the park, I read our city map and noted the name – Slottsparken, or the Palace Park. It was where the Royal Palace was. There was a lot of scaffolding up on the outside of the palace. It seemed as if extensive renovation work was going on. The palace looked down on to the main boulevard of Oslo, called Karl Johans gate. I came to realise that the word '*gate*', when combined with one or more other words, meant the name of a street.

I came across a royal guard outside a sentry box. The guard stood out because his skin colour was so black. I was surprised. We were in Scandinavia and I expected to see pale skin, blue eyes and blonde hair everywhere. I thought, I must look up something about that later. I liked the way he looked and wanted a photo with him. 'May I have my photo taken with you, please?' I asked him. He said nothing but nodded ever so slightly. Sue took a photo of us with me on my yellow scooter. (Photo 3.1.1)

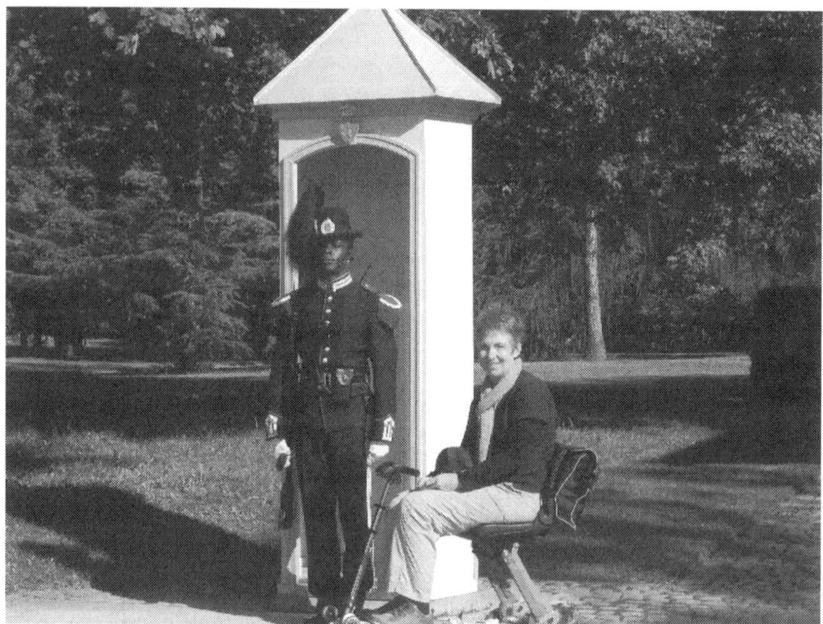

Photo 3.1.1 On my scooter with a palace guard in Oslo

The day was beautiful, with blue sky and sun shining on green grass. We enjoyed being in the park and took some photos and videos of trees, the lake, statues and other royal guards. It was very easy scooting around the park; there was level access everywhere. My first overseas adventure with my yellow scooter was going very well.

On the way to the park, we stopped and bought two filled bread rolls. We sat in the park later on and ate the rolls, watching Oslo go by. It was nearly 2 p.m. when we headed back to collect our keys.

The charge in my scooter was getting low again. After a full charge, the instruction manual said it could go seventeen kilometres, or about three hours for me. That was without stopping, on level ground. However, the earlier charging session at reception had lasted only an hour or so and a full charge took longer than that. I was still learning about the battery. When I was at home, my outings didn't take many hours at a time and were all on flat ground. Going up inclines used more power and the battery ran out faster.

I waited on my scooter near the side street where our apartment was to save the battery while Sue walked all the way back to Frogner reception. If we got stuck, we could roll it down the hill from there, I thought.

There was a very busy road at the top of our street. I was on the footpath of Drammensveien. I learned later that it was a highway between the cities of Oslo and Drammen. There was a lot of traffic, but it didn't feel like a highway.

The sun was still out and I enjoyed getting some more Vitamin D. I was opposite the park, next to a restaurant with an outdoor area spilling on to the footpath, and a bicycle rank. It was nice just sitting there on my scooter watching what was going on all around me. I may have been in a bit of a daze by then. Every now and then, I stood up to stretch my stiff legs and move them about.

Sue came back with the keys and a bit of grocery shopping that she'd done on the way. I'd noticed quite a few fruit and vegetable shops in that area as we'd gone past before. The owners all looked as if they came from Middle Eastern backgrounds. They displayed their fruit and vegetables outside, perfectly and beautifully arranged in open sloping wooden shelves. I'm sure Sue noticed them before me, and she probably wondered what was different and new to us and what was fresh.

We went down the street to turn into Arbinsgate and down again to our street number. There was a glass door opening off the footpath with three small steps to get up inside. Then there was a level entrance area, before … I couldn't believe it … a long set of steps! About twelve steep steps going up. The stairs went up to another landing with more glass doors. The lift up to the other floors was on the other side of those doors, up that flight of stairs. Fredrik's 'three small steps' at the beginning was correct but it certainly wasn't step-free after that!

There were no apartments off that first lower entry level. We soon discovered that our apartment was at the next upper level, immediately after the twelve steep steps, through a solid door to the right. We didn't need to use the lift, positioned where it was, behind the next set of glass doors. It was no help to us.

I felt disappointed with Fredrik and the poor information he'd given me. But, oh well, what could I do now? It was the end of a long day. I was tired. I just had to deal with it.

I left my scooter at the entry before climbing the twelve steps. I went up the steps one by one. I thought I'd only really need to do this once or twice a day so I'd just have to manage. Up at the next level, through a heavy fire door on the right, was a corridor leading to several apartment doors. Ours was the second one.

I spotted a free power point near the entry before the stairs. We thought we'd leave the scooter there, off to one side, to happily charge overnight. It shouldn't be in anyone's way and it was safely locked behind the entry door.

The apartment was big enough, with a lounge area and an open kitchen off to one side. The dining table was elevated and ran off the wall. You had to perch on a bar stool to sit at it. That wasn't ideal for my legs. The bathroom had a tiny step up into it and the shower had semi-circular round opening doors surrounding it. It looked all right to stand in.

The bedroom was roomy and the beds nicely made. All the floors were wooden, a little minimalistic and bare. There were two windows, one in the lounge and one in the bedroom. They looked out on to an enclosed cemented courtyard. It was all a little unusual but we thought it would work out okay. I got around it easily using just my walking stick.

We unpacked a few things and then I had a rest while Sue went off to find a supermarket. When Sue arrived back, she said, 'I found a small one nearby. I asked some people where a larger supermarket was. I don't know if they understood what I meant. I've bought a few things, though.'

'Oh, good. Show me, please.' Sue had bought some good basic provisions – breakfast cereal, pasta, a pack of smoked fish, some fruit and vegetables.

'Someone said there was another supermarket down the street the other way. But I didn't know where they meant.' That was something for the next day. Sue cooked dinner as she always did and I washed up. The meal was good and healthy, and we went to sleep not long after. It had been a long first day, but we'd settled in very nicely.

We were going to spend four more days in Oslo. We wanted to do a lot of walking and get a real feel for the place. We woke up the next day, raring to go.

The first thing that struck me about walking and scootering on the footpaths in Oslo was the number of drains that went across them. Drains from roof gutters came down the sides of buildings and the water came out at right angles into troughs across the footpaths. The gutters were part of the top of the path, open and not buried under the concrete as in Australia. One came out from every house. They were made of multiple segments that fitted neatly together. Every ten metres or so, my scooter wheels had to go down and up a few centimetres to get over them. It wasn't a smooth ride. I tried going slowly, but that didn't make it any easier. I stopped a few times to take drain photographs.

An early stop, down the hill and over the drains, was at the local tourist information office. It was near the Rådhus (the town hall) and the waterfront, exactly where we wanted to go first.

It was cloudy weather today. Then it started to rain. It rained on and off from then on for most of the time we were in Oslo. Sometimes it varied in heaviness. That first day of sunshine was the one and only sunny day we had. We had water-resistant jackets and pants, with hoods on the jackets to pull up and over when the rain was heavy. There were very few umbrellas up; people were just out in jackets. We joined in.

The tourist office was behind the town hall and some way back away from the waterfront. A vintage car event on the waterfront drew our attention. The Akershus Castle was up behind this gathering of cars.

A banner read '*Norsk Veteranvogn Klubb*'. We walked around and looked at the old cars. There were ones that reminded each of us of our past cars, such as my VW Beetle and Volvo. Some of the people there were very interested in my scooter. They watched it go by and eyed it up and down. Maybe it was because they'd not seen a scooter like it before or maybe it was because it was bright yellow. I've had many people tell me they liked my scooter. 'That's something!' they might say.

We decided to walk back into the centre of town and down Karl Johans gate. Despite the weather, the city was full of people. They were sitting in cafes, riding bicycles, walking and shopping. There were vertical banners everywhere that said, '*Universitetet i Oslo 200 år*', letting people know there was a University of Oslo commemorative event that week. The university was at the top of the street, just down from the Royal Palace and the Palace Park. It was two hundred years old, only forty years older than the universities of Sydney and Melbourne.

We wandered down towards the central station, checking out the cathedral on the way. Scattered around the cathedral were flower wreaths. They were left over from memorial ceremonies held for the victims of the shootings a few months before. It was as if the people of Oslo were still coming to terms with what had happened.

A little further along Karl Johans gate was a market with lots of stalls. Then I saw it – a beanie with ear coverings. Just what Raina had recommended for the cold. I found one with a bright pattern and plaited ties to fasten under my chin. Written on a tiny label were the words '100% Wool, Made In Nepal'.

The cap was made of two layers and the knitted outside was plain-stitched using different colours of wool. The wool smelt and felt greasy, like a natural untreated fibre. Funny, I thought, to be in Norway buying a Nepalese beanie. Nepal was in the Himalayas. Wool comes from sheep, but I didn't think there were any sheep in the Himalayas. Then I remembered that wool also comes from yaks. The beanie must be made out of yak wool. The stallholder didn't speak English, but I smiled and was very happy to hand over the equivalent of AUD$10. As I left, he nodded his head and smiled too.

We moved on and found the central station. I wanted to

investigate the location of our hotel accommodation on the last night, right at the end of our trip. It was the Thon Hotel Opera and it was right beside the central station as the website indicated. Then we saw the Opera House beside it too. Wow! What a wonderful piece of architecture. We went straight there to look more closely. We took lots of photos and videos. I loved it.

The newly constructed Oslo Opera House was like an iceberg on the water, all white and reflective in stone and glass. It was magnificent. It sloped upwards, at first gently and then steeply, out of the water. I stayed down the bottom and took photos. Sue walked up to the top and took videos along the way. She waved from the top and I took a photo of her waving arm with my superzoom camera.

We went inside the Opera House and that was amazing too. The walls to the open cloakroom were lit up and made of multiple protruding pieces. They looked like origami coming out of the walls. I asked at the ticket office about seats for an opera while we were there in Oslo. They only had one ticket left in an accessible area on the dates we were there. I wouldn't go on my own. I thanked the woman and declined. Another time, I thought. It would have been special, though, in that wonderful venue. That was something else to book before leaving on another trip.

We went back to our apartment, taking a different route. We stuck to the waterfront this time. There was a lot of building and restoration work going on. The pathways weren't easy. After a while, we crossed the road and headed into the old city area. Finding our way around barricades and detour signs, we suddenly came across two young women. One was lying on the ground; she was just a young teenager and she didn't look well. I was about to offer to help when I saw that the other girl was helping her inject something into a vein in her arm, which had a tourniquet around it. Oh, what a shame, I thought, so young and taking drugs.

We were the only other people there and it was getting late. We moved away and headed home. We walked through parts of the old city where there were various art galleries, but none seemed open that day. They didn't seem to be easily accessible, anyway.

We ended up back near the tourist information centre on the harbour. The Nobel Peace Centre was there too. We earmarked it for another day.

As we were coming back up the hill to our apartment, we suddenly saw it, a large sign on the outside of a building, which read 'Vinmonopolet'. It was the liquor store Raina had told us about. The building was a brick, three to four-storey, office-type structure with no windows. We ventured in and discovered it was a small shopping centre. Vinmonopolet was only one shop of many in it. There were three floors of all sorts of shops, including a good-sized supermarket. We went into Vinmonopolet first.

There were so many wonderful varieties of wine to choose from. They came from all around the world, including Australia, just as Raina had said. We wandered around enjoying ourselves. Sue was in seventh heaven. She has a very good knowledge of wines. At one stage in her life, she was thinking of doing a degree in oenology at Roseworthy College in Adelaide. I thought some of the wine labels must have brought back wonderful memories of other places she'd visited.

Sue soon spotted a friendly sommelier. They had a conversation and, before long, he was recommending some good French and Italian wines at reasonable prices. We started our wine adventures in Oslo with one bottle of white, one of red and a sticky.

Carolyn had warned us about the price of wine here. 'We all joined AA for the three weeks,' she said. They hadn't heard of Vinmonopolet, and we were so grateful to Raina.

The supermarket was the next port of call. 'Meny' the sign read. That was its name. Meny was much the same as supermarkets at home – except the labels weren't in English! But the pictures on the packets helped a lot. The goods for sale were similar to products at home. Everyone there had a similar appearance to us as well. I didn't feel foreign. No one seemed surprised to see me on my scooter.

Finding plain rolled oats took some time. There were many different types of grains and cereals. We'd made a few mistakes in the past when we were away, getting flour instead of oats, for example. I kept the Meny supermarket receipt and made a copy with my translation alongside it. (Photo 3.1.2)

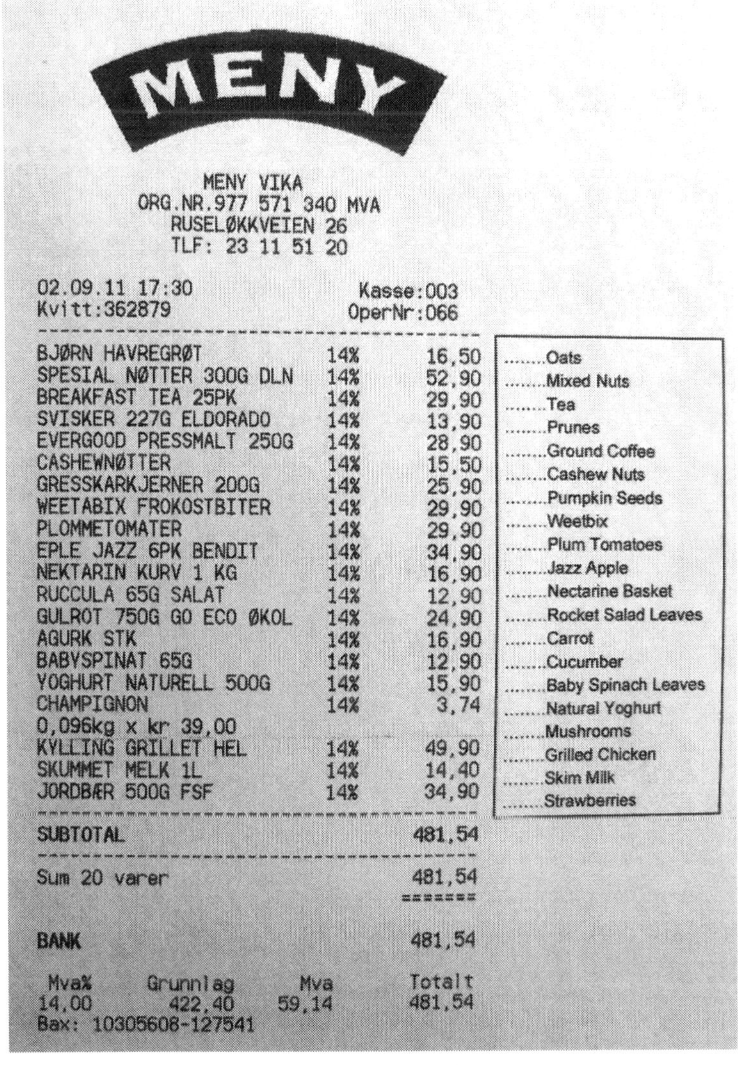

MENY

MENY VIKA
ORG.NR.977 571 340 MVA
RUSELØKKVEIEN 26
TLF: 23 11 51 20

02.09.11 17:30 Kasse:003
Kvitt:362879 OperNr:066

Item	Mva	Price	Translation
BJØRN HAVREGRØT	14%	16,50	........Oats
SPESIAL NØTTER 300G DLN	14%	52,90	........Mixed Nuts
BREAKFAST TEA 25PK	14%	29,90	........Tea
SVISKER 227G ELDORADO	14%	13,90	........Prunes
EVERGOOD PRESSMALT 250G	14%	28,90	........Ground Coffee
CASHEWNØTTER	14%	15,50	........Cashew Nuts
GRESSKARKJERNER 200G	14%	25,90	........Pumpkin Seeds
WEETABIX FROKOSTBITER	14%	29,90	........Weetbix
PLOMMETOMATER	14%	29,90	........Plum Tomatoes
EPLE JAZZ 6PK BENDIT	14%	34,90	........Jazz Apple
NEKTARIN KURV 1 KG	14%	16,90	........Nectarine Basket
RUCCULA 65G SALAT	14%	12,90	........Rocket Salad Leaves
GULROT 750G GO ECO ØKOL	14%	24,90	........Carrot
AGURK STK	14%	16,90	........Cucumber
BABYSPINAT 65G	14%	12,90	........Baby Spinach Leaves
YOGHURT NATURELL 500G	14%	15,90	........Natural Yoghurt
CHAMPIGNON	14%	3,74	........Mushrooms
0,096kg x kr 39,00			
KYLLING GRILLET HEL	14%	49,90	........Grilled Chicken
SKUMMET MELK 1L	14%	14,40	........Skim Milk
JORDBÆR 500G FSF	14%	34,90	........Strawberries

SUBTOTAL 481,54

Sum 20 varer 481,54
=======

BANK 481,54

Mva%	Grunnlag	Mva	Totalt
14,00	422,40	59,14	481,54

Bax: 10305608-127541

Photo 3.1.2 Meny supermarket receipt

The 481.54 Norwegian kroner appeared later on my credit card statement converted to Australian dollars. The supermarket items cost AUD$83.64, not including a currency conversion fee of AUD$2.51. We'd bought breakfast for the days we were in Oslo and more things for lunch and dinner.

I noted the fourteen per cent GST. Other European countries had a much higher rate. In Australia, it was ten per cent. It was interesting to see how other countries managed their finances.

The apartment was closer to the big supermarket than we'd realised. We'd been shopping in a different direction at a small corner store. The Meny supermarket was much better. Some of the load fitted into the backpack on my scooter seat. Some light things fitted in the little pack on my back. Sue had the heavier backpack and bags to carry by hand. I suppose we looked a bit funny all loaded up.

For dinner that night, we had grilled chicken with salad (rocket and baby spinach leaves, plum tomatoes, cucumber, carrot and mushrooms) and some of the wine Sue had chosen. We followed that with fresh fruit (apple, nectarines and strawberries). Very nice, I thought.

Dinners on the other nights were often composed of pasta with a tomato-based sauce, served with salad or vegetables. It was easier to stay at home at the end of the day, especially when it was dark. Riding the scooter in daylight, looking ahead frequently for anything that it might not be able to negotiate, took enough concentration. In the dark, it was harder. I didn't want to roll the scooter over and injure both it and me. It was healthier to eat at home too; as Sue said, 'We know exactly what's going into that meal.'

The apartment kitchen had an electric stovetop with hotplates, and there were pots, pans and other cooking implements in the cupboards. Sue would cook and I'd wash up. It felt a bit like home. I found washing up physically much easier to do than cooking. I'd lean on the sink while I washed; I could stand like that for at least ten minutes or so. Cooking was much more difficult and I wasn't very good at it either, unlike Sue. Our division of labour in the kitchen worked out very well for me.

We had plenty for breakfast too. There was cereal (oats and Weetbix) with prunes, pumpkin seeds, fresh fruit, natural yoghurt and skim milk, followed by plunger coffee served black. The breakfast tea we'd bought was for an afternoon cuppa if we found ourselves back at the apartment for a rest and recharge (of both me and the scooter).

We tried to watch some news most days. We'd settle down with a glass of wine and a few nuts. It took a while to find the right television station to watch. We wanted to see the local weather reports for the next day. At the end of the thirty-minute news, there were weather maps. It looked as if there were morning and afternoon reports for the days ahead, along with some helpful symbols. The sun symbols didn't last long. We could see cloud and rain symbols over most of southern Norway, especially over Oslo, on the days we were to be there.

I'd borrowed Carolyn's Gore-Tex jacket with a hood for the trip. I wore it every day for warmth and against the rain. It was wonderful to have it. I had a cheap clear plastic fold-up poncho ready to put over everything as I rode my scooter, but I never used it. Sue wore my Snowgum water-resistant jacket and occasionally an old red rainproof top with a hood. That was better for her to walk in. I had another borrowed item, a set of black wet-weather Mont waterproof pants as well. My friend Barb had leant them to me to go to Antarctica and I still had them. Barb had said she'd found better ones for her long holiday walks and gave me the Mont's. My legs were warm and waterproof with her pants on over my lightweight travelling pants, especially with thermal underwear underneath. The clothes we'd packed were working out well.

We wanted to catch the boat across to the Bygdøy peninsula to visit the Kon-Tiki Museum and the Viking Ship Museum. Carolyn had sent me a photo after her trip; she was wearing the black jacket and standing in the rain waiting for the ferry. We hoped the weather would improve before we ventured there ourselves.

I did think to myself that we could always get a taxi. Sue must have read my mind. She said, 'Let's just go down to the dock and check out the ferry. It should be a good way to get there. I cannot remember how I got there thirty-five years ago.' Sue didn't like taking taxis when there were better ways to experience a place.

'But what about after we get there? There's a bit of a walk, isn't there? So the book says.' I answered, thinking that might convince her. I didn't mind taxis.

'Oh well, we won't be the only ones walking. We'll figure it out,' said Sue. She'd always loved walking.

We left the apartment and went down the hill. I went over the drains across the footpaths again, bumpity bump, every few metres. I went ahead and Sue walked behind me. I heard Sue call out from much further behind, 'Oh, look at the baby!' I turned and went back to Sue, who was looking down a space between two buildings to a small, shared backyard. There was a large, light grey and white, very good-looking cat, sitting upright very neatly and looking straight at us. 'Oh, hello baby. What are you doing?' Sue asked.

Looking for the sun, I thought. I took a photo of the cute furry feline, with its two front paws placed together, looking into my lensed eyes. Some of the flowers blooming in the sheltered courtyard helped make it a very pretty picture, I thought. We didn't see many dogs or cats about in Oslo. That was interesting too.

There really wasn't much sun that day, and the rain, light at first, suddenly came down in waves. We went full speed down the hill and bought tickets for the ferry. Sue asked for directions to the museums. I could see big ferries coming and going. The access on to them looked easy – I'd just have to wheel straight on and in across a wide ramp. We asked people coming off if this was the right ferry to get to the museums. We didn't get a definite answer. Perhaps our communication wasn't clear.

I waited in the rain and Sue went back to the ticket office. She soon came back. She was pointing and saying, 'It's further around on that other pier over there.'

Our ferry was tiny. It looked like it would take only a dozen people. But it was the Bygdøy ferry. There was an old wooden ramp with crossed boards. The dockhand beckoned me forward.

I bumped over the ramp and into a small area next to the captain. There were steps down after that. I stayed on the top level. It was a little under cover. I hoped it would be a beautiful trip on the fjord (our first one), with city and mountain views. It was misty and rainy but I could still see some things as we went out into the harbour and headed south-west.

We disembarked at a small pier with a tiny shed in among a few houses. It looked like we were on the edge of a residential suburb. Houses were neatly dotted along the street. There were no signs to give us directions. But there was only one street, so this must be the way to go, we thought. Off we went. There was a footpath but it was narrow. Occasionally, I had to scoot out on to the road. There was no traffic, anyway. It was cold, misty and a bit dark. There was a wintry feeling and no people were around.

There was a sign at the end of the road, which indicated that the Kon-Tiki Museum was quite a few kilometres to the left, and only two kilometres to the right to get to the Viking Ship Museum. We went right.

I was starting to feel a bit miserable. I was a little wet and a bit tired from negotiating my way along paths and roads in those unpleasant conditions. I was starting to feel cranky with Sue that we hadn't just got a taxi in the beginning. That would have been much easier, I thought, and I wouldn't feel so bad.

Sue took a video of me going along to the front entrance of the museum. People have told me they can read my face like a book. I can't hide how I feel and I can never lie. My face was turned the other way for the video, thank goodness!

I had no real idea of what the Viking Ship Museum was. I thought there'd be parts and replicas of some of the old Viking ships used in this part of the world centuries ago. When we arrived there, a tourist bus had just arrived and people were pouring in. There was hardly any room to move. A rope was blocking the entry to a striking-looking Viking ship. There didn't seem to be anything else there. There were steps up to view the ship from a higher level, but no ramp or lift for me to get up there.

There was a ticket office to one side and a queue. Everyone from the bus had some sort of pass. Another busload arrived. We took a few photos from outside the barrier and left without ever going in. Anyway, I was most interested in photographing the curling shape at the top of the bow of the ship. It looked like an unfolding fern branch. I wanted to catch its shadow on the wall.

It wasn't until we went to the museum at the University of Oslo – the Historical Museum – a few days later that we realised what we'd failed to appreciate and what we'd missed. I felt very silly. They were burial ships! In Egypt, I'd oohed and aahed at the burial chambers with their jewels, gifts and furnishings. All those articles, buried with a person to take them through to the next life. Pharaohs were buried in pyramids and in secret enclosures in mountains. Viking kings were buried in a similar way but in ships. I had no idea at the time. The ship with the curling feature extending out from the bow was the Oseberg ship – the most important piece of Viking history there was. And we went in and out in under ten minutes!

After we came out of the Viking Ship Museum, I didn't think my scooter battery would last the distance to the Kon-Tiki Museum and home again. It was too far. The weather still wasn't pleasant. Then we saw a bus stop. We asked the people waiting there where the bus went. A couple explained that they were going back into the city, to the left.

Then an older man said, 'A bus will be here soon. Another bus should come and stop on the other side of the road, down there.' He pointed to his left.

My map showed a bus route going past the Viking Ship Museum from the city and then turning right. It looked like it must go past the Kon-Tiki Museum. The rain had stopped so we waited where the man had pointed. The people at the first stop caught the bus going to the city and a few minutes later a bus came to where we were waiting.

Sue and I discussed how we'd get the scooter on board. We wouldn't know what kind of bus it was until it arrived. We'd just have to deal with it – and we did. I got on and Sue lifted one end of the scooter up, rolled it on to the bus beside the driver's section and sat down. About fifteen minutes later, we got off at the Kon-Tiki Museum.

The Kon-Tiki Museum housed the famous raft sailed by Thor Heyerdahl. He was born in 1914 and died in 2002. He was one of history's most famous scientists, adventurers and environmentalists. The *Kon-Tiki* balsa raft journey was a historical experiment. No one believed his theories, which took him ten years to research. The scientific community told him his ideas were not plausible. He had to personally re-enact his theories to prove they were true.

In 1947, Heyerdahl and his crew of five men travelled from Peru to Polynesia. He showed that people from early South American civilisations could have reached Polynesia with seafaring vessels some 1,500 years ago. Winds and ocean currents could have carried them.

The Kon-Tiki Museum housed original vessels and exhibits from many of Heyerdahl's world-famous expeditions. The museum was home to permanent exhibitions about the *Kon-Tiki* as well as his other vessels, the *Ra* and the *Tigris*, and his expeditions to Fatu-Hiva and Easter Island. In the same year of our visit to the museum, Heyerdahl's archives became part of UNESCO's 'Memory of the World'.

I found the rafts and reed boats fascinating. It was hard to believe those materials could float. The huge single oar rudder used at the back of the boats and rafts to steer them was something I'd never seen. There were small huts on board some of the vessels too. People had lived in them for months. They were exact replicas of what were used thousands of years ago. I took many photos because I was in awe of what had been achieved. And that way I could prove that I saw it!

After the Kon-Tiki Museum, we went across to the museum opposite. It could have been a Viking ship construction museum. The entrance into the building was closed, so we couldn't go in. I was hungry by then, anyway. It was well into the afternoon and I still felt a bit wet too, and a bit miserable. I just wanted to stop for a while. We had bread rolls and cheese in the backpack so we sat at the water's edge and ate them. The bay, the harbour and the fjord were very peaceful. It was quiet, the sky was filled with grey clouds and some mist. After about twenty minutes rest, I felt better and ready to go again.

We found another museum nearby, the Polarship Fram Museum. We had to visit it. After all, the name of our cruise ship was the MS *Fram*. Inside was the actual old ship with three open viewing floors built up around it. There was also the story of polar exploration, north and south. Australia received more than a mention. We spent a lot of time at the museum, reading about Amundsen, Shackleton and other polar expedition heroes.

The bus stop was back outside the Kon-Tiki Museum. We knew the bus stopped there and I'd noted that it took a circular route. We'd already been on part of that route. We walked back and only had to wait a short time before the bus came.

I noticed that the bus had a wheelchair accessible sign on it and realised that I probably needed to alert the driver so that he could stop the bus close to the footpath. I thought that might allow him to put some sort of ramp down for me. I'd seen one of those coming out of a bus door before, in Honolulu. The driver had got up and lifted a ramp down for me on my blue electric wheelchair. Here, in Oslo, the bus stopped out on the road and no one got out to work the ramp, so we made our own way out to the bus.

We put the scooter on the same way as we did before. Once on the bus, we went down to the middle where there was an open area with no seats and another door. There was plenty of room there for the scooter and there were free seats either side of it.

It was a local bus and it felt good to be surrounded by locals on a regular timetabled route rather than on a tourist bus. The suburbs and houses were interesting to see and I enjoyed listening to banter in another language.

When we reached the familiar central Oslo area, in the distance I saw an elevated tram and bus stop across the road from the top of our street. I pointed it out to Sue. Ours was the next stop. I looked around and realised there were three large baby prams surrounding me. My scooter was smaller than the prams. It usually was. I turned the scooter on and indicated that I was moving to the door. There was a fast kerfuffle of men parking prams and offering to help. Sue started to pull on a ring in a metal plate on the floor by the doorway. Oh, I thought, that's how the ramp works. You pull it up and fold it out and then down. But the ring broke off in Sue's hand. She was standing in the bus with a large ring in her fingers, laughing. Messages were passed up to the front of the bus to let the driver know he had to wait. It seemed as if he was about to move on and we weren't yet off.

In situations like this, I've learned to get off my scooter quickly, move to the door with my walking stick, and get out and wait. Sue looks after the scooter or supervises the helpers. There were quite a few men helping this time. We were off and the bus nearly took off again with one of the men outside and his baby in the pram still on board. There were shouts inside the bus and it stopped. The man went back in amid cries of thanks from both of us.

We went down the hill to the Meny supermarket, Vinmonopolet and then home.

That night, when we were watching the news on TV, Sally Pearson appeared on the screen. She'd just won the women's one-hundred-metre hurdles at the 2011 World Championships in Athletics in South Korea. Wow, what a wonderful achievement! We both made impressed noises – they were reporting an Australian achievement here in Oslo!

One day, when it was raining heavily, we decided to stay indoors as much as possible. We got the umbrella out this time, covered up, walked and scootered to the museum associated with the University of Oslo, the Historical Museum. It was in an Art Nouveau building near the Palace Park. It only took us about ten minutes to get there.

At the main entrance to the building, there were two sets of stairs going up to the front door. There was no wheelchair or disabled access to be seen and no sign to say where there was one.

'I'll go up and ask how you can get in,' said Sue and went up the stone steps to get inside the museum. I pulled my hood over my head and tried to shelter from the rain under a tree.

When Sue came back she told me, 'We have to go around to the back of the building. There's a goods entrance there and someone will meet us.' We went around and couldn't see anyone. We knocked on an old door and, a few minutes later, a male security guard and female museum worker came out to greet us. The woman apologised about the lack of accessibility and for not being at the door sooner. They took us up in a rattly goods lift, escorted us along some dark and dusty passageways and then took us through a door into the museum. We went through a medieval collection of stave church doorways, sculptures and paintings into the main admission area. No wonder it took them a while to get there, I thought!

The Oslo Historical Museum opened to the public in 1904. It houses about 1.5 million artefacts collected over two hundred years. It holds all sorts of antiquities.

There were four floors with ten permanent exhibitions. On the first floor, we learned about the Vikings' lives and saw some of their ornaments, tools and weapons. These were on the same floor as the 'Ice Age to Christianity' exhibits, which showed aspects of people's lives from the Stone Age to the Middle Ages. In this last section, as well as tools, there were sacrificial finds, gravestones and burial gifts from prehistoric times. In between these exhibits was the 'Treasure Chest'. It contained a collection of gold and silver jewellery and other valuables, including Norway's largest gold treasure from Viking times, the Hoen hoard.

To get to the other floors in the museum you have to use a large central staircase. So I went via the goods lift with a security guard again.

My favourite area was on the second floor where there was an Arctic and Subarctic exhibit. It would be only a few days' time before we'd be north of the Arctic Circle ourselves. It was all very new to me. There were displays of traditional clothing, tools, equipment, and arts and crafts from Greenland, Siberia, Northern

Canada, Alaska and Lapland. I'd never seen anything like it before.

While we were on that floor, one of the museum guards came up to us and said, 'Come over and have a look at this.'

We went with him to a tall glass cabinet with a mannequin dressed in something unusual.

'See, this long coat, it is made of fish skins sewn together,' the guard said. He explained some of the customs of the indigenous people of the Arctic.

It was fascinating. The fish-skin coat was almost transparent. It served as a loose outer protective layer worn over other clothes. The clothing was all made from natural materials – skin, fur, bone and other animal body parts. People used whatever was available to them in that hostile environment.

We went past some exhibits from America and saw a bead-embroidered child's vest made by the indigenous people of the Great Plains. It was a long way from home. We left soon after, because we felt we'd been there long enough. After an hour or so, my brain stops absorbing information. We were satisfied with what we'd seen.

We did, however, go to the museum's coin cabinet before we left. One of the rarest coins on display was Olaf the Holy's penny, from 1015. I thought its name was interesting and that it was worth a quick look.

While we were looking at the coins, I turned the museum brochure over and discovered some information about the Viking Ship Museum. I said, 'Sue, look at this! This is where we went the other day. They were burial ships. Look at all the things that were there. And other ships too. We just saw this one, here, the Oseberg ship.' I pointed to the picture in the brochure. 'We missed a whole lot of things.'

Sue looked at the brochure. 'Oh dear! We need to read that tonight.'

We went out on to Karl Johans gate and looked for a coffee place. We saw a sign that said '*Kaffebrenneriet – Stedet for God Kaffe*'. 'Kaffebrenneriet' was the name of the type of place where we'd had our first coffee, near Skovveien 8 and the Frogner reception. This place had to be good too. I took a photo of Sue in front of the sign so I could remember our good coffee spots.

The cafe was packed. There was no room to sit down or scoot in. I'd read that Norwegians drank more coffee per capita than any other nationality. We couldn't fit in.

I'd also read about Stockfleths, an award-winning cafe, and one of the oldest coffee shops in Oslo. It was supposed to have good bread and sandwiches too. We went down Karl Johans gate. I had a city map on which I'd marked spots for good coffee that I'd heard about. Distracted by the wonderful shops on the way, we didn't make it to Stockfleths or any of the other spots I'd noted. Instead, we found an okay-looking cafe tucked at the back of an arcade of shops. There was a disabled toilet nearby. Perfect, I thought.

I recalled being in a small shopping centre a few blocks away on another day in Oslo. The sign to the disabled toilet indicated how to get there; it was via the lift. I waited outside the lift on my scooter with an older man and his severely disabled son, who was in a wheelchair. We waited together for a while and then we both realised the lift wasn't working. We exchanged a frustrated look. I felt lucky; I could scooter off quickly to find somewhere else. This man had to wheel his son's large wheelchair much more slowly. I wondered why they didn't build all the disabled toilets on the ground floor.

On our way back home that day, I thought about the next stage of our journey. I was keen to have a clear plan in my mind for getting to the airport. It would be early in the morning on the day we were to fly to Longyearbyen to start our cruise. This involved investigating the lift situation at the train station. As it turned out, there were two parts to the investigation.

When we arrived in Oslo, we got off at the Nationaltheatret stop. There were at least three exits from that station. The one we chose on the day we arrived was the one furthest away from our apartment. When we'd got a better feel for the place, we noticed two more Nationaltheatret entrances. One was up the street and across the road from our apartment, under the Palace Park. The other entrance was on the same street but down towards the shopping centre on the same side as our apartment. They were both underground, with varying distances to get to the platforms.

The fast train to the airport, the Flytoget, shared Nationaltheatret Station with other trains. The Flytoget route was on one line, with trains only going to or from the airport. The silver Flytoget trains were more modern and faster than the other metropolitan and regional trains.

The train platforms were underground and serviced by lifts and escalators. We had an early flight requiring an early start, and I thought it would probably be raining again too. We definitely needed the shortest and closest route from our apartment.

I found that we had two short options to choose from to get to the station platforms. I wanted to see them both first-hand so I could check their accessibility and see which platform was the right one for us. So, at the end of the day, on our way home, we walked and scootered the routes. We chose the one near the shopping centre to start with.

At the entrance off the street was a revolving glass door for wheelchair users. It seemed different to the ones back in Australia, which are bigger, slower and a bit scary. I always feel I might get caught in them somehow. But I went in and out of the ones in Oslo on my little yellow scooter with no problem.

Sue opened the glass door and went down the stairs. I took a long ramp down and away from the platform entrance. After going down the ramp, I went back along the lower level to meet Sue. We checked out the ticket machine, the ticket office and the noticeboards for departures. Then there were two choices to go down to the platform on the next level. One was an escalator. The escalator's moving staircase was not suitable for wheelchairs or scooters. The other choice was a lift. We chose the lift and went down one level on to the platform.

We watched a Flytoget train come in and leave. They went often, it seemed. Then we walked and scootered down to the other end of the same platform. That led to the second way in and out of the station, under the park. There was a well-lit and gleaming escalator, and a lift from the platform up to the next level.

Then, oh no! The lift seemed to be out of order! Nothing happened when we pressed the button. I just had a feeling that something was wrong. I waited at the bottom while Sue went up the escalator to check our theory.

I watched a woman come along the higher level with a pram; she attempted to use the lift. A man with a suitcase came close behind her. They seemed to be in a hurry and weren't happy that the lift wasn't working. I guessed they must have been trying to go to the airport! Everyone seems to be in a rush when they're going to airports.

The lift didn't work and they struggled to get everything down the escalator. A Flytoget train came and went. That was a bit of a lesson, I thought. I took some photos of the escalator and lift as a memento and waited for Sue to come back.

'Yes, that way goes out to the entrance under the park,' said Sue when she got back. 'I think we'll use the other entrance on the day and take the lift that we know is working. We won't risk it.'

I certainly agreed. We went back the same way we came in to go home. We felt very pleased with ourselves for finding out so much useful information. As it turned out, the events at the station on the day we had to travel were much more dramatic.

At some stage during our stay in Oslo, we went to the main tourist information centre. We went to the one at the central station. Apart from information about Oslo, I asked about the train in Bergen – the one we had to catch to do the Nutshell. I also asked about the ferry and the bus. Yes, there was a problem with the line but the train I'd booked should be okay. The assistant wasn't sure of the details of the bus at Gudvangen, but there was one, and he said the ferries were still running at Flåm. He suggested I enquire again in Bergen.

While we were at the information centre, my scooter battery indicator light showed that the battery was very low. I spotted a free power point in the wall. Since owning the yellow scooter, I've developed a knack for spotting an available power point. I usually try to find one in a coffee shop. I rode my scooter over to the point and plugged the charger in.

There was an espresso coffee machine in the centre. It was definitely time for a coffee, a stretch, some leg exercises and a seat in a normal chair. The coffee was surprisingly good. We rested there for about an hour and read the tourist brochures we'd collected.

By then, both ourselves and the scooter were rejuvenated so I unplugged the charger and put it back into the pack on the back of my scooter seat. We headed off.

I thought I couldn't be in Oslo and not visit the Nobel Peace Centre so we went there next. There was so much to see, do and read at the centre.

I was astounded when I came across a photo and the story of Mairéad Corrigan on the second floor. Back in late 1976 and early 1977, I went on my first overseas trip. I went to the United Kingdom and over to Europe and back. I decided not to travel to Ireland because of the bombings and shootings associated with her name. She was in the news so often – the famous Miss M. Corrigan. That's my name too! People had made death threats against her. I really wasn't sure if she was a good person or a bad one at the time. I just knew that the IRA was involved and it wasn't safe to travel to some places in Ireland. My gut feeling was that she was probably a good person, but I didn't ever find out.

Here she was, in a photo in a room upstairs at the new Nobel Peace Centre in Oslo. There were time periods set out on a wall with the names of the people who had received the Nobel Peace Prize alongside. A brief story about them was set out on a digital touch screen. Mairéad Corrigan was a Northern Irish peace activist. Born in Belfast, she co-founded the Community of Peace People, an organisation dedicated to encouraging a peaceful resolution to the troubles in Northern Ireland. Mairéad Corrigan received the Nobel Peace Prize, together with Betty Williams, her fellow co-founder, in 1976. She was a good person. I felt very proud of her.

After the Nobel Peace Centre, we decided to wander further down the waterfront and along the harbour's edge. The old seaport was being rebuilt. There were ferries loading and unloading passengers and, just beyond that, there were wonderful views looking back to Akershus Castle, with ships, boats and ferries in the foreground. We admired the view, took a few photos and videos and kept walking.

The Aker Brygge, a complex with big shopping centres and restaurants, was just there too. We decided to just note them and walk past. There seemed to be more to see beyond that area.

We soon came to a very new area called Tjuvholmen. Construction of that area began in 2005 and it was due for completion in 2014. The brochures called it 'Oslo's trendy quayside'. There were apartments, offices, shopping areas and hotels, as well as art and culture venues. The architecture was very modern and I liked it. There was a lot of glass in odd but good-looking shapes, and some of the buildings seemed to flow into the water while others leapt straight up and out. I took many photos, but it was dull and rainy weather; I didn't think they'd turn out to be as good as the real thing.

Soon, it was time to go up the hill and home. We tried to go a different way every time. Today, a huge, haunting building on a hill near our apartment caught our eye. Perhaps I was in an architecturally appreciative mood or perhaps it was the dull, bleak sky in the background that made it stand out.

It was Victoria Terrasse, the headquarters of the Gestapo in Norway from 1940 to 1945, after the Nazi invasion. I'd forgotten that they were in Norway. Apparently, at the time, Victoria Terrasse was known as *skrekken hus*, the house of fear. I later read with great interest about the Norwegian Resistance and their courage during World War II.

I like to think that if I were put in that situation, I'd have chosen to be a resistance fighter. Perhaps that's some oddly romantic view of mine. The outside of the building itself looked fearsome, never mind what went on inside.

We bought some groceries and more supplies from Vinmonopolet and went back to the apartment feeling very grateful to be in Oslo in the year 2011 and not in the 1940s.

On our second-last night in Oslo, the weather reports seemed to say that the next day might be the best for some time. When we woke, it did look as if it might be sunny at times. So we decided to go to Vigeland Park. Mum had told me about the park and its sculpted figures, and so had Raina. It was sort of on the way to the ski jump at Holmenkollen and that was also on our list of things to see.

We wanted to take one of the newer accessible trams the man at the Oslo tourist information office had spoken about. We hadn't caught a tram in Oslo yet, though we'd seen them about. We found the tram stop nearest to our apartment on the map and went there.

One tram came by and then another. They were all old ones with two steep steps up to the seats. When the next one came, Sue went up to the driver and asked him how long he thought it would be before the accessible tram came. The driver said that none of those trams ran on this line. But he got out from the tram straight away and helped Sue lift the scooter up the steps and inside.

When we arrived at the Vigeland Park stop, the tram driver helped us off. He was just matter-of-fact, courteous and helpful. It was no big deal, it seemed. We went across the road and into the park.

The park was huge – many acres in size – and there were many sculptures of naked human bodies of all ages and sexes. These granite, wrought iron and bronze sculptures were the work of the Norwegian Gustov Vigeland, who lived from 1869 to 1943. His works showed people displaying every possible kind of emotion. The theme was the human condition, and the park was the world's largest sculpture park by a single artist.

There were many people out walking, playing, sitting and chatting. In particular, I noticed two elderly women, one with a walker and the other with two walking poles. They were walking side by side, chatting as they moved slowly along together. I thought they looked wonderful making their way enjoyably through the park. I watched them for a little while and they struck me enough to take several photos.

All the paths were accessible and flat except for one area around a tall, round sculpture that looked like a monument. There were a lot of steps up to see it and what was sculpted around it. I waited at the bottom of the steps and looked in the opposite direction. That's when I first noticed a very large ski jump on a mountain behind the park. When Sue came down, I pointed it out to her and we went over to the edge of the park to get a better look. What a structure! It was impressive.

After walking and scootering around in the park for a little while longer, we headed off to the ski jump. I assumed that the one I saw in the distance was the one we wanted. We went in the direction of a metro train stop that was clearly shown on my map. It was only a few blocks away. But first, before catching the train, we needed a coffee. We stopped at a place in a small shopping area near the train station. A sign said they roasted their own beans, so we thought the coffee there had to be good. And so it was.

I needed to stop and stretch again as well. I could only sit for about an hour at a time on the scooter. The muscles in my legs would start to feel stiff after that. I needed to stand up and do some exercises to move my legs about. I also liked sitting in a normal chair whenever I could because it was easier to move my legs while I was seated and I could do a few different exercises. I stood up, did some exercises standing and then sat in a chair at a cafe table and moved my legs a bit more.

***

'Spasticity' is the proper name for that stiff feeling. Sometimes it feels the way I used to after doing unaccustomed exercise – after playing a game of squash when I hadn't practised for a few weeks or the feeling the day after walking many kilometres without doing any training. It was an interesting name, spastic. I've heard that word used in conver-

sation in the past to mean many different things. I once looked up the word's origin. It's derived from the Greek word spastikos ('drawing in' or 'tugging'), meaning an alteration in muscle tone.

I feel stiff a few times each day. It isn't pleasant so I suppose it would qualify as pain, but I don't think of it that way. Standing up and moving usually helps, but sometimes I just have to say, 'Oowww... Ooorrhh... Urrrh,' and that takes people by surprise if I don't remember to say it quietly. So I suppose it is painful, after all, that stiffness.

***

After my stretching and exercising, we both sat and watched the world go by for a few more minutes. Then we were off again.

We went to the local metro station and started to purchase a ticket. Then we remembered that we'd bought a two-day travel pass when we caught the ferry to the Viking Ship Museum. We were still within the two-day period, and the pass covered all forms of public transport in Oslo. We just waited for a train on a platform with a 'To Holmenkollen' sign. A train arrived quickly and we got on.

The train had level access from the platform into the carriage. However, the gap between the platform and the floor of the train was too wide for me to ride my little yellow scooter over. The wheels were too small for the gap. I got off, we folded the scooter down quickly and I stepped on. Sue followed with the scooter. She struggled a bit to get the scooter in, and a man on the train came over to help her.

The man looked at the scooter as he was helping Sue and noticed my name on a label on top of the battery. I'd stuck it there in case the scooter ever got lost. He said 'Maureen Corrigan... Is that the same Maureen Corrigan who...'

Sue pointed to me. He looked at me. I looked at him.

'Graham! Hello,' I said.

'Yes,' he said. 'We used to play tennis together at Gosford! Do you remember?'

'Yes, I sure do.' That was over forty years ago! On this particular train, on this day, at this time, in this country, I run into somebody I haven't seen for many years. He was my mixed-doubles tennis partner in what was then country NSW, at the local Brisbane Water Tennis Club competition. We played every weekend for years, until I was sixteen years old and went to boarding school in Sydney.

He was living in Perth, Western Australia now. He had come over to Norway with his wife to visit their son, who lived in Oslo, and have a holiday. They were also on their way to the Holmenkollen ski jump.

We chatted – mostly I answered his questions – and I missed all the scenery as the train climbed the hill. Graham said their son had told them about a great restaurant just below the ski jump that had wonderful views. They were going to have lunch there and invited us to join them.

The scooter battery was running a bit low after all the kilometres it had done. When we arrived at the restaurant, I saw there was a steep climb up to the ski jump. I asked the waiter at the restaurant if I could plug in my scooter to charge somewhere out of the way while we were having lunch. 'Yes, of course,' he said, and showed Sue where to take it.

The four of us talked over lunch. The food was lovely. Just one main course was perfect. The view was wonderful even though I had my back to it at the table. After lunch we headed off up the steep hill to the ski jump. I'm not sure if Graham had intended going any further than the restaurant, but I indicated that it was a must-do for me.

I took Graham and his wife's photo for them in front of the Holmenkollen ski jump sign and then went up the footpath. When it ran out, I went on to the road. It was very steep and I wasn't sure if my scooter would be able to manage such an acute angle. I was still learning about that side of things. But my little yellow scooter proved its strength and we went up the steep hill slowly but without any problems. I leaned forward to help us along.

The ski jump was enormous. I'd never seen anything like it before. The images of ski jumps in the Winter Olympics were of those covered in snow. This was just after the end of summer. We could walk up to the halfway point. No snow anywhere. Gee, it was steep!

I bought three postcards of the ski jump from the gift shop. I sent one to Mum because I thought it would strike her fancy and she'd mentioned a big ski jump in her old postcard. The other we sent to a friend and I kept one to go on the fridge back home. (Photo 3.1.3)

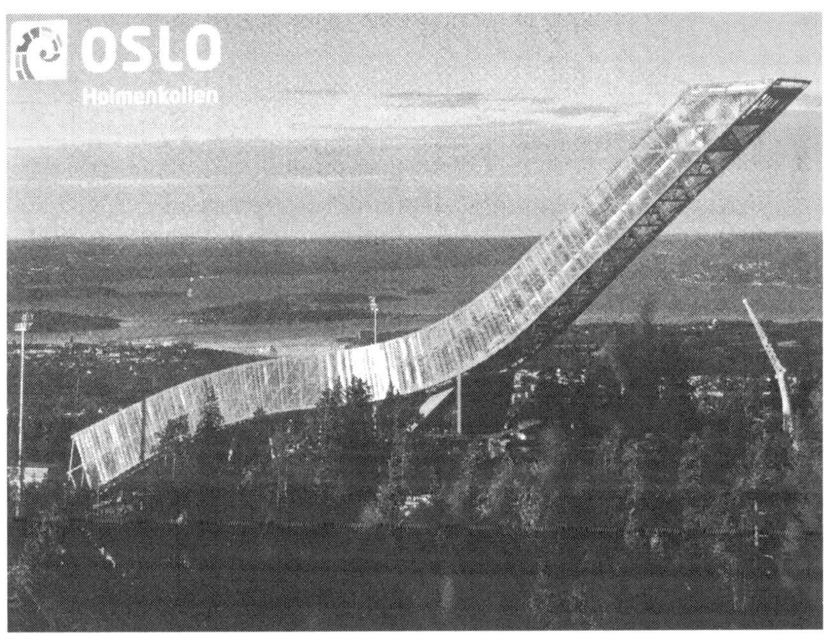

Photo 3.1.3 Holmenkollen ski jump
Image credit: Photo Normanns Kunstforlag

I agree with Mum about getting postcards. Postcard photos usually had the best images, taken from the best perspective under the best conditions. Sometimes I'll look at postcards in a shop to give me an idea of how best to take a photo of a place. I couldn't take a photo from anywhere near the perspective of the one of the ski jump. It was taken further up the hill at quite some height, I thought.

Near the gift shop, at the halfway level of the ski jump, there was a building with a glass wall. Behind the glass wall was a room with a large, moving capsule in it. I could see a person inside the capsule; a sign said that the movement simulated the ski jump experience. You had to be in good control of your balance to be able to try it. I'll certainly do some daring things but I said no to that one. My MS had made me more sensible.

***

My MS affects my balance. It's probably one of the main reasons I need a four-wheel walker. It's to stop me falling over by giving me something to hang on to.

Sometimes I don't have to hang on to anything but I do have to touch something. A wall is often good to touch as I move from one room to another. Sometimes I find myself standing in one spot, unable to move away from the wall because I've left my walking stick somewhere. I have to think where I might have left it and retrace my steps back along the wall. I feel a bit silly at these times; my mind was obviously elsewhere when I took off.

Balance issues can arise from problems in the cerebellum at the back of the brain. When I've read my MRI scan results in the past, I've seen that there are MS lesions in my cerebellum. Good, I thought then. I have a reason for my balance problems.

***

There was supposed to be a museum up that hill. We looked but we didn't see it. Soon, the weather was closing in again; there were dark clouds overhead and all around us. We thought we'd better get out of there. It would be steep-going down that hill and I didn't want to skid, slip and slide in my scooter.

We reached the train station at the bottom of the hill where we'd got off only a few hours earlier. There were modern, brightly coloured apartment buildings built to one side of the station. They would have looked out over the station, down to Oslo one way and up to the ski jump the other way. They looked attractive. I took a photo of them while we waiting to catch the train back down to the city.

Graham and his wife went to the ticket machine at the other end of the station and came back with another woman. There were only about four other people at the station altogether. When the woman came up to us, she said, 'I thought I recognised the accent!' She was well-spoken and had a slight Australian accent. 'I'm from Melbourne originally, but I live here now.' She pointed to the apartments on the other side of the station.

We all explained where we were from and why we were in Norway. Then we caught the same train down the mountain to the city. I sat with the woman, whose name was Ann, and we started to talk about the issue of disability. Ann explained that she was interested in how riding horses assists people with disabilities. Ann was writing a thesis. I was very interested in what she had to say. Ann went on to talk a little about her working background in health. The conversation became even more interesting.

Before too long, Ann and I realised that we had a connection. We'd both worked with the same people at some stage. Some of those people were also now friends. What a very small world it was, I thought. On this train, at this time, I had Graham over on the other seat from the 1960s and Ann working with the same people that I'd worked with in the 1990s. All that happened in Australia and here we all were in Oslo, Norway.

I didn't get to see much of the view on the way back either. So there were no scenic photos taken on that train trip, but there were many good memories revisited. We each got off at our stops, said goodbye and continued on with our plans. Our stop was the now very familiar Nationaltheatret.

It was our last day and we'd planned on going straight home from the station. We were just up the hill from our apartment when I noticed the Ibsen Museum. It was around the corner from our apartment. I said, 'I really think we should see this. He was a famous writer, wasn't he?'

'I think he wrote plays,' said Sue. 'All right. We're here now. Let's see it.'

The next hour or so was wonderful. We were lucky to be there when a tour of Ibsen's home was about to start. He'd lived in that building, upstairs in an apartment. There was now a modern lift from the renovated ground floor and mezzanine levels of the museum up to the first floor.

After we arrived on level one, the tour guide told the group which way to go and then took me on an alternate route so I could avoid the old narrow corners, passageways and doors that my scooter wouldn't have been able to negotiate. There were two other people on the tour and we all met up again at the entrance to Ibsen's apartment.

The building was on a street corner. One street of the corner was ours – Arbinsgate. The other was the main street that we'd walked in from. It was named after him – Henrik Ibsens gate.

The apartment had been restored to the way it was while Suzannah and Henrik Ibsen lived there, in a way that was true to the decor of the time. It also contained Ibsen's own furniture. This was where he'd lived for the last eleven years of his life, from 1895 until his death in 1906. The passionate tour guide told us, 'He wrote his last two dramas here, *John Gabriel Borkman* and *When We Dead Awaken*. This is where he sat and wrote, and this is where he looked out on to the park, through this window.'

The guide told us that Ibsen's presence at the window was a popular attraction. People walking past would look up to see him. I felt it was a privilege to be there and to see the private sphere of Ibsen's life during his later years. The furnishings were beautiful; he must have been quite wealthy by that stage in his life.

I was amazed by the small size of his bed and his bedroom. His wife had her own small bedroom too. Ibsen had a single bed, which stood against the wall, with carved wooden ends. I didn't know how he, an adult, had fitted into it. Photos of him showed that he wasn't a small man, either!

After looking through the apartment, we went to the museum on the mezzanine floor. There was an exhibition on called 'Henrik Ibsen – On the Contrary'. It showed the kind of person and playwright that he'd been. Some of his personal belongings were displayed there as well as much of his writing. The exhibit said that it showed 'the dynamic power of Ibsen's drama' and shed 'light on his political views and their relevance to national and international issues'. I didn't realise how outspoken he'd been on the rights of women. I liked that.

I later learned about some of his more familiar plays, *Hedda Gabler* and *A Doll's House*, in which he told stories about women that were quite different to the conventional views of his time. He shocked people by portraying women as independent, and challenged the norms of gender at the time.

The Ibsen Museum was the last place we visited in Oslo. The next day, we were going to fly to Longyearbyen to start our expedition cruise.

We organised everything so that straight after breakfast and the washing up, we could walk straight out of the door. I hoped it wouldn't be raining and I hoped that we'd get to the airport in plenty of time.

I was starting to worry a bit about all the rain falling on my battery. The water might get into the connections between it and the scooter and then the scooter might fail. I'd been happily scootering around in the rain just about every day, but when I started to think about how important it was to get to the airport I came up with a method of covering the battery to protect it. A plastic bag with an old piece of newspaper over the top would do the trick, I thought.

We left early the next morning in light rain. I posted the ski jump postcard to Mum in the red postbox at the street corner on the way down to the Nationaltheatret entrance. It was about 6.30 a.m. The newspaper over the plastic bag seemed to be working well to cover up my battery.

Through the revolving doors at the station I went, and then down the ramp to meet Sue at the bottom of the steps. We'd bought our tickets on our practice run days before. That was the time when the lift at the other entrance wasn't working. But, this morning, the lift at *this* end wasn't working! It was hard to believe. I said the obvious to Sue. 'It was working the other day! It was the other lift that wasn't working, not this one. This one was okay then. So much for all the checking!'

There was now a sign on this lift saying 'Out of Order. For Assistance Go to Ticket Office.' When we went there, there was a sign on the ticket office too. It said 'Closed'! Only the escalator was working. Perhaps the lift at the other entrance might be working now, I thought. But it would take too long to get there – we'd have to go out, up the hill, across the road and under the park. I'd allowed about thirty minutes extra for the whole trip to the airport in case there was a problem. But I thought that going that way might take even longer than that, and the lift might still not be working when we arrived there.

There was an office upstairs. Sue saw it. Off she went and I scooted around and went up to help. Sue knocked on the door and a man in a uniform opened it. I could see that it was a security office with a one-way mirrored wall around it. There were many video monitors on desks and hanging from the ceiling. One person could sit and see what was going on all around the station. Sue told him the problem and asked for help. He said he was on his own and couldn't leave the office.

Sue pointed at his big, weight-trained arms and said, 'A muscly guy like you should be able to lift that little scooter up and carry it down the escalator in no time at all. It only weighs twenty-three kilograms. It won't take long.'

He took up the challenge quickly and we all headed back to the top of the escalator. I got off the scooter and the security guard lifted it up and carried it down. Sue followed with the suitcase. I still had my little backpack on. I had my walking stick and intended to grab and hold on to the handrail of the escalator. I wasn't worried about getting on as much as I was about getting off at the bottom. Sue was ahead, ready to help. On I stepped and down I went. A few people were rushing past to get ahead. That was also the last thing that I needed. I wanted a clear spot at the bottom. I made it and stumbled only slightly. Sue had the security guard there, ready too.

We were okay. We were on the platform and had ten minutes to spare. The sign above read 'Flytoget, Oslo Lufthavn/Oslo Airport'.

The fast train was taking us back to the airport at Gardermoen. The flight from Oslo to Longyearbyen was included in our cruise package. It was with Scandinavian Airlines and left from the same airport at which we'd arrived.

There were no problems at Oslo Airport and I remained on my scooter all the way from check-in to the departure gate. I sat in the waiting area of our gate lounge and watched the activity around me. Men and women were moving around on large push scooters. They had one leg on a wide plank on wheels and pushed with the other leg. They were picking up and delivering cardboard boxes to the shops on the concourse. Their scooters were very quiet, but fast. I'd never seen them before. What a great idea, I thought.

I spotted a disabled toilet over in a corner while we were waiting to board. It was fantastic. I could reach the button to open the doors automatically and it was big and clean. But I did have to wait my turn outside. After quite a few minutes, a good-looking young man, very nicely dressed and with very neatly combed hair, came out. He was *not* in a wheelchair. He looked at me sheepishly as I went in.

Back in the departure lounge, I suddenly noticed how light and bright the terminal was. There were big windows, open spaces, high ceilings and woodwork in that light Scandinavian birch colour.

Oslo was a good place and a very enjoyable one to visit. After five days there – it seemed much longer – I felt I'd got a real feel for the place. We saw and learned so much. My yellow scooter had worked out reasonably well in its first overseas city. We'd had to lift it up a few times to get into buses, trams and trains and we hadn't had to do that before. But its small size made it manageable and, yes, the three of us had managed it all very well. A few interesting dramas had taken place, and even a big one while getting to the airport!

When it came time to board and have the airport staff collect the scooter, we collapsed it down and Sue tied one more strap around to secure it. An attendant brought a wheelchair and I transferred into it. We boarded early, first as usual, with two other people in wheelchairs. We all went into the covered air bridge and on to the plane. We left on time at 9.55 a.m. on Scandinavian Airlines flight SK4414, on Wednesday, 7 September.

The flight over the coastline of Norway had fantastic views. There were islands, mountains, rocks, raised lakes, snow, sea and bays. We landed in Tromsø first for security and passport checks. We were staying in Norway for the whole trip so I wasn't sure why we had to land there. No one else seemed to know either. At least we didn't have to disembark.

I thought it worked out really well, though, because as we were flying in to Tromsø I saw a large bridge over the waterway close up. It was the same bridge that I'd seen in postcards back in Oslo. I could take my own photo and I did. Tromsø Airport was close to the bridge and it was a spectacular sight to see on landing.

The total flight time of our trip that day was four hours. We didn't have to sit in the plane at Tromsø for very long at all. We were soon in the air again and heading north-west, away from the Norwegian coast and towards the North Pole. We were going to start the next phase of our trip.

CHAPTER 2

LONGYEARBYEN AND THE SHIP

The plane landed at Longyearbyen in the early afternoon. I looked out of the window and saw that it was raining. I also saw two wheelchairs parked at the foot of the stairs leading up to the aircraft. Straight away, I remembered that three of us had boarded the aircraft in wheelchairs and suspected something not good was about to happen. I took a photo of the wheelchairs just to be able to tell the story later. There was not a third wheelchair in sight. From where I was sitting, there was also no lifter that I could see.

The other two, much older, people who came to the plane on wheelchairs ended up leaving on the two wheelchairs that were waiting. What I suspected would happen did happen. I explained to the aircraft crew that I had difficulty walking, trouble with stairs, had booked a wheelchair and that I needed one too. I said that I had to get to the baggage area to get my own 'wheelchair'. That didn't make any difference to the situation. They were not forthcoming in offering a solution or help.

I was the last to leave the plane. There didn't seem to be any other way than to just try and get down the stairs and walk what looked like seventy metres to the terminal. It was still raining. So I struggled down the stairs on to the tarmac.

After only a few metres, I was already walking with great difficulty. I had my walking stick in one hand and the other was holding on to Sue's arm. An airport attendant came up and said, 'This is not right. Wait here and I will go and get one of the wheelchairs that are in the terminal. There might be one free by now.'

By the time the wheelchair arrived, I'd reached a wall and was leaning on it with great relief. I waited a little while and was soon in the available wheelchair. They had found another one.

When I was finally inside the terminal, I saw the other two people in wheelchairs get up, collect their bags and walk away. They were both older than I was but they could walk a lot better. From outward appearances, they might seem to need more assistance than I did. This had happened before. I must just look too young – and too well! I was still in my fifties and I looked quite capable. But I'd booked a wheelchair too. I did feel annoyed.

A local guide was waiting in the arrivals area holding up a sign. My scooter had arrived safely and in good order, together with our luggage bag. We were with a small group and the guide took us out to a bus. The bus had a cardboard sign on it that read in large print 'MS *Fram*'. Everything was loaded on to the bus and we drove off. The rain had stopped by then and I'd calmed down after the wheelchair mix-up. Seeing my yellow scooter arrive safely always reassured me. And now it was tucked away in the luggage compartment, not far from me at all.

We were in the Svalbard, a group of islands – an archipelago – in the polar north. We were 650 kilometres north of mainland Europe and still in Norway. Longyearbyen was the biggest of the three towns in the Svalbard. With a population of about two thousand people, Longyearbyen was located on the bay of a fjord on Spitsbergen, the largest of the islands. The islands of the Svalbard formed a gateway to the permanent ice sheets covering the North Pole, and Longyearbyen was the closest large settlement to that pole surrounded by sea.

As we were flying over Longyearbyen, I remembered once watching a documentary on TV about the Global Seed Vault. This underground vault, built in 2007, was a secure site to house seeds from across the world in case there was a global catastrophe. The vault was in a permanently frozen mountain just north of

Longyearbyen. The view from the plane looked the same as it did in the documentary.

As we flew over the town, I could see that it sat at the base of a crescent of snow-covered mountains. A waterway formed a neat line for the plane to fly over before it landed at the base of the mountains, at the town tucked into the crescent. That was the same sight I'd seen on television. I was excited about being there, seeing the real thing, and I thought I must keep an eye out for the Seed Vault.

There was snow high up on the mountains and the roads around the town were made of paved bitumen with stone and gravel along the sides. Longyearbyen reminded me a bit of a ski resort in summer. There were low-rise buildings of one, two or three levels raised off the ground. They were all different colours, with plenty of Ski-Doos parked outside.

The bus took us all to a hotel in Longyearbyen not far away from the airport. We were going to spend the night there and board the ship the next day.

A sign outside the entrance to the Radisson Blu Polar Hotel explained that it was customary to take off your shoes and leave them on the shelving provided.

There wasn't far to go on my scooter from the bus to the hotel. There was a raised piece of wood running along at ground level at the hotel's entrance. It was too high for the scooter to go over from the bitumen outside. After the strip of wood, there was a thick, brushy mat and then another wooden strip, and finally the hotel carpet. There were two sets of doors too, but they were both open. I thought the entrance must have been designed to keep the snow, ice and mud away from the inside, and the brushy mat was there to remove any excess that made its way in on shoes. This was all new to me.

Sue and I lifted the scooter wheels over the first bump. Then we dragged and pushed it slowly to the next bump and lifted it over that one as well. Other people from the bus were making their way around us. I thought they looked at us, wondering what we were doing. Someone offered to help but we were just about through by then. We were managing all right on our own even though it was a little difficult.

'Thanks, but we'll be okay,' I said.

Once I was back on my scooter and on the carpet with clean wheels after going over the mat, it didn't make any sense to take off my shoes. They weren't on the floor. They hadn't been in any mud. Sue took hers off and wore socks inside the hotel.

Our room had a thermometer outside the window. It read 5°C. I'd expected it to be cooler but I was pleased it wasn't. It was afternoon and our tour schedule said that after check-in it was a 'day at leisure'. We thought we'd go for a walk into the main part of the town. We put on coats and lifted the scooter back over the front entrance bumps again. Sue put on her shoes as we went out past the shoe shelves.

Outside, we went down the hotel driveway, over a road with no traffic and on to a wooden boardwalk. This took us over some permafrost soil and vegetation and on to a bitumen footpath into the town centre, which had its own smooth bitumen areas surrounding the shops, offices, post office and school. It was easy-going on my little yellow scooter. The tallest building in the town was two storeys high, but most were only one-storey and were easy to look into.

There were some shops grouped together, including a small clothing shop with Arctic knitwear on show. There was a polar bear on a sign outside with the word *Svalbardbutikken* above the bear and 'Longyearbyen 78°13′N' below it. I thought the first word was the name of a boutique store; to have one this far north seemed special.

It became very cold very soon. A strong wind developed and I understood the term 'wind-chill factor' – I could feel it straight through to my bones. We quickly went in to what looked like a supermarket, where there was a ramp for my scooter. After that, there were two low bumps and two sets of doors wide apart. I could easily ride through if Sue held each door. Oh, it was warm inside – lovely!

The store was a large general store with food items at one end and clothes and other goods at the other end. The cash registers and exit areas were just like those in our supermarkets at home. We checked everything out and bought some postcards. The receipt also said *Svalbardbutikken*; the sign I saw outside was referring to this big shop. My Norwegian to English translation was not correct at all. *Butikken* just means 'shop'. I also noticed from the receipt that all the goods sold here were tax free – no GST. Interesting.

We noticed quite a few people looking around the alcohol section and we stopped briefly to look at the wine labels. Then we braced ourselves for the walk back to the hotel, which was only about four hundred metres or ten minutes. We stopped at the post office for stamps (with polar bears on them), which was a good opportunity to make sure we had all our zippers done up and cords pulled tight.

For dinner that evening, we went to the hotel restaurant, the Nansen, named after the famous Norwegian Fridtjof Nansen (1861–1930). Nansen was the inspiration behind the original polar ship, the *Fram*. There was really nowhere else to go for dinner. The other choice would have been to buy some dinner supplies at the supermarket. Dinner was not included in the package deal but we decided to splash out on the first night.

We went to dinner and it seemed funny for Sue to be wearing just socks on her feet. I parked my scooter and walked to the table with my stick and Sue's arm. My shoes were on my feet. I couldn't walk comfortably in just socks. I needed lace-up shoes with a stiff sole to help counteract my left foot drop.

***

That foot drop – an inability to lift my left foot properly – was my first symptom of MS. At the end of my daily thirty-minute walk first thing in the morning, I started to notice that my left foot was making a floppy sound as it hit the footpath. For a little while, I just thought I was unfit or had been working too hard and not getting enough rest.

Then, on bush walks, I started to trip over towards the end, and the flopping sound was happening more often.

One day in 2001, after a bush walk and a fall after tripping, I sat in the passenger seat of my car and realised I couldn't lift up my left leg. I felt nothing. It just wouldn't move. I thought, Oh dear, this isn't right. I need to see someone about this. Over the next hour or so, the weakness in my left leg and left foot went away and I could walk again. It was the weekend, but as soon as Monday came I made a few phone calls. I saw a neurologist soon afterwards.

At the time, this weakness came on only with exercise. I recovered when I stopped. I learned later that my body temperature needed to cool down. Then a few other odd things started to happen. My left hand didn't have the same dexterity as it usually did. I noticed this for the first time when I was using the keyboard on my computer. This episode – of what I learned much later was MS – lasted a few months. After that, I felt fine for some years.

Then my MS progressed. And now, in Norway in 2011, some ten years after I'd first developed foot drop and sought help, I was using electric wheelchairs indoors and walking short distances with other aids. I read somewhere that twenty-five per cent of people with MS could be using a wheelchair within ten years of diagnosis. But I also read that the percentage is dropping because of the new immunomodulating drugs, such as Tysabri.

The fact that some of my symptoms get worse with exercise and then go away after rest, is something about my MS that I find very interesting. I read a lot about my symptoms and MS in the early days after I was diagnosed and, from time to time, since then.

The first piece of information about foot drop that I read was in relation to Uhthoff's phenomenon. I found the information in Harrison's Principles of Internal Medicine. Uhthoff (1853–1927) was a famous German professor of ophthalmology. In 1890, he discovered that a temporary loss of vision could occur in someone with optic neuritis following a hot bath or exercise. A patient of his complained of going blind when she was in a warm bath; she would completely recover a short time after she got out. Similarly, some people suffered temporary loss of vision during exercise. Uhthoff was the first person to describe the phenomenon, which was later found to be caused by a rise in body temperature. Further work showed that other neurological symptoms could also become worse with exercise because of an increase in body temperature. My foot drop is one of those neurological symptoms.

I'm one of the seventy-five to ninety-five per cent of people with MS who are heat sensitive. After too much warming exercise, my left leg can become completely paralysed. It also becomes difficult to think properly when I'm hot. Everything improves when the temperature around me, and my body, cools down. I've learned to limit my exercise to twenty minutes and to avoid warm baths, pools and hot places. I've also adopted a whole range of techniques to keep myself cool.

I once tried using an ankle-foot orthotic device on my left leg. The device held my left foot up and stopped it from dropping, dragging and scraping as I walked. But, after a few years, I found that the device was preventing me from bending my ankle and that it was no good for going up an incline. I also found the device heavy and irritating so I stopped using it. A firm shoe with a strong sole was good enough.

***

We sat in the dining room, eating local fish and looking out at the fjord and the spiky mountains that gave Spitsbergen its name. It was spectacular. The food was good and the wine was okay too!

Our instructions for the next day were to have our luggage ready early in the morning and to place it in the luggage room dedicated to MS *Fram*. The ship departed in the afternoon and bags had to be put into the cabins before departure. Our instructions also said to attend an information meeting at the hotel. Our shipping service Hurtigruten posted a notice at reception to say the meeting would be at 10.30 a.m. in one of the hotel's large rooms.

Further instructions said there was a 2 p.m. pick-up for a bus tour of the town and the island. We'd then arrive at the pier at 5 p.m. Sue and I had to think about what was ahead of us the next day, what we were going to wear and when we'd wear it. My scooter wouldn't be luggage that early, though, as I'd still need to ride it.

The next morning, we went to the information session and a member of the Hurtigruten team presented some details on the cruise ahead. I introduced myself after the thirty-minute talk. I was sitting on my scooter. I asked, 'Is there anything in particular I should note because of my mobility?'

'No, I don't think so,' was the reply. There were no special instructions.

We also had to hand over our passports at the meeting to clear immigration and customs during the voyage. The team said that the ship's officers would keep the passports in a safe place until the end of the trip.

We noted that the bus planned to leave the hotel after our usual lunchtime. Lunch was not included in the package. We'd have to get our own. We wanted to go for a longer walk around Longyearbyen anyway. We went out via the supermarket again and bought some nice cheese and bread. Then, off we went to see more of Longyearbyen on our own. There were no footpaths, but there weren't many vehicles moving about so we went on the roads. The few people we saw were all walking on the roads.

The scenery was unlike anything I'd ever seen before. There were old mining structures scattered about on the lower parts of the mountains. That was their 'cultural heritage', a travel brochure said. Buildings, coal-mining equipment, large buckets on chains held by rails on posts, gantries and other buildings used to mine, transport and burn coal at small power stations were all lying about. The buildings and structures were still standing exactly as they had been on the day that operations ceased. That was decades ago, and the metal had rusted. It was quite a scene, especially with two glaciers as a background. Later, I read in a brochure that 'any pre-1946 remains of human activity are classified as "cultural monuments" and aren't to be touched'.

The Svalbard Museum was located away from the town centre, down near the water of the fjord. There was a visit to the museum on the afternoon bus tour, but we thought we'd go on our own, to have a better look without a crowd. On the way down the road, I only had to pull over on to the gravelly dirt a few times for passing traffic. We went past a shop selling ski gear and another shop selling reindeer and sealskins. There were small trucks loading and unloading goods outside. One or both businesses must be thriving, I thought.

Further down the road, we saw a large sign on a building with two sections. It read 'Svalbard *Forskningspark*'. Below that, over an entrance to the left was another sign that read '*Universitetssenteret På* Svalbard' and '*Norsk Polarinstitutt*'. There were a few other signs on the right as well.

Although I didn't get *butikken* right, I thought I could work out most of what the signs were saying because the words seemed very close to English. I thought that the signs on the left meant that a university department and institute were located there, while on the right, the signs clearly indicated the Svalbard Museum and the Tourist Information Centre. But I had to ask about the word *Forskningspark* later. It meant 'research park'. I took a photo of Sue under all the signs because I wanted a record of the correct spelling. That was another reason I took photos.

Once inside the museum, shoes came off again. This time there were Croc-like plastic shoes to put on. They were in all different colours and you just had to find your size. Sue put the Crocs on and I stayed on my scooter Croc-less. Then we had a leisurely time looking around the museum and reading various pieces of information. It gave us a good idea of where we were, where we were going and the history of Longyearbyen.

The museum visit finished our self-guided walking tour and we ate our lunch of bread and cheese outside in the sun before going back to the hotel to wait for the bus.

We loaded on to the bus as scheduled and my scooter went into the outside bottom luggage area. First stop was another hotel.

I realised that the passengers for our cruise were coming from different places at different times and days. This hotel was where the other half was staying. Then there were two buses. One bus was for Scandinavian and English speakers and the other for German speakers. There was a short break at the hotel while things were organised.

Then we were off to do a brief tour of the town and the immediate area, with a few stop-offs included to visit local galleries and the museum.

We went to the art and craft galleries first and then drove out of town past a large residential area. The buildings, painted in different colours, were in blocks. Many of the blocks were two storeys tall with ten to twelve units in them, and there were about thirty different blocks. There were also some individual houses linked to each other directly or by covered passageways. The blocks of units lay parallel to each other in steps going down the side of the hill. To me, it looked like a combination of a ski resort and an industrial camp.

Soon after leaving the town of Longyearbyen on the only road north, the colours on the ground hit me. I looked out and across the expanse of land to the jagged mountains behind, and the green and yellow shades were amazing. I kept taking more and more photos. The colours of the low-lying vegetation were beautiful. Some plants grew close to the ground, tiny and delicate. There were miniature grasses, little flowers and lichens everywhere. Sometimes the ground looked pink. It seemed to be a truly colourful Arctic wilderness.

There were reflections in the low-lying water. These reflections of mountains and grasses were in one of the postcards I'd bought. I tried to take a photo like the one on the postcard, but the sun wasn't out and the conditions weren't the same. The photographer was probably better too! I tried to capture some of that colourful vegetation at Longyearbyen in the foreground of my photo. (Photo 3.2.1)

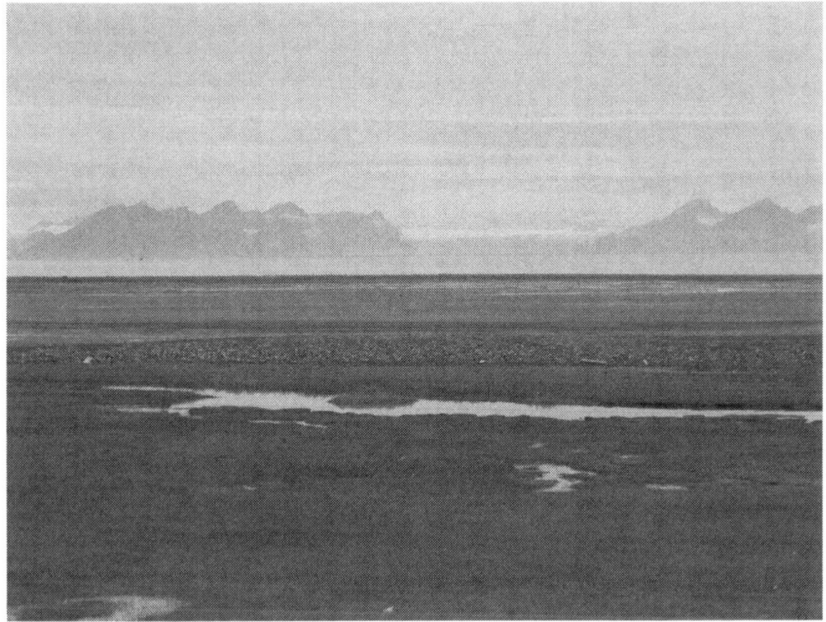

Photo 3.2.1 Colourful vegetation at Longyearbyen

Some of the reflections in my photos were of the mountains and some were of the old mining sheds and equipment. The latter looked odd but also beautiful.

But the actual scenes of 'cultural significance', without the reflections, weren't beautiful and weren't what I was prepared for. The buildings and equipment left standing or falling down to age naturally undisturbed, looked to me like uncared-for industrial rubbish. Their setting and scale was different to anything I'd ever seen. Probably like something my mother would call a 'one off', with a meaning quite different to mine.

Our bus drove past a large pound of husky dogs. They looked healthy and barked loudly as we went past. They each had their own kennel elevated high off the ground. Wire fencing surrounded the sides and wire also ran across the top of the whole area. I could imagine those dogs pulling sleds in the snow very efficiently.

The buses arrived at a sign that seemed to indicate there were polar bears in the area and to be wary. Everyone got out of the buses without hesitation and took photos of the warning sign and the surrounds! (Photo 3.2.2)

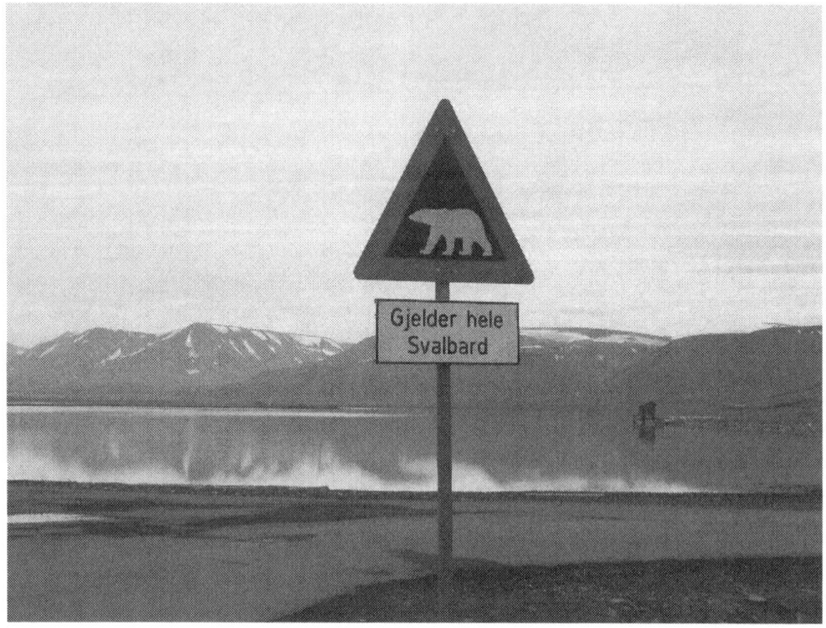

Photo 3.2.2 Polar bear warning sign

The buses turned back after that and we stopped at the Svalbard Museum back in town. The museum was very crowded with the people from the two buses. It was especially crowded at the front entrance where everyone had to change shoes, except me. I was pleased that we'd visited earlier. Still, there were other things to look at and read the second time around. It was a good museum and I learned even more about the town and its coal-mining industry on that second visit.

The name Longyearbyen comes from John Munro Longyear. He was from the USA, and started coal mining in Spitsbergen in 1906. He established the Arctic Coal Company. German marines largely destroyed the mining town in 1943; it was rebuilt after World War II. Today, tourism and research are growing and mining has mostly moved to other sites on the island. Longyearbyen is still the base for the workforce but now they fly in and out of the other sites in shifts. That was probably why I didn't see too many locals about.

Longyear City was the town's original name. It changed its name later to Longyearbyen. I looked up the word *byen* later. It means 'town' in Norwegian.

After the museum, it was time for the bus to go on to the other side of town where there was a cemetery and a church on the side of the mountain. The historic graveyard had simple white wooden crosses in it. Seven men were buried there. They died during the 1918 worldwide flu pandemic. That influenza virus, known as the Spanish Flu, infected five hundred million people in the world and killed fifty to one hundred million. It came this far north as well.

We drove past the Svalbard church building. Our guide told us that it belonged to the Church of Norway, and was used for both religious and cultural activities. It was the northernmost church in the world. The Church of Norway had its origins in the Lutheran Church.

Our guide was a young woman who spoke in alternating languages, first Norwegian (I thought) and then English. I said to Sue, 'Gee, she speaks English well.'

Towards the end of the tour, when we were up the front of the bus, we thanked her and complimented her on her ability to speak two languages so well, especially English.

'Oh, I was worried that my Norwegian wasn't good enough,' she said. 'I've only been learning it for a short while.' She spoke with an Australian accent! She added, 'I come from Brisbane. When I was speaking on the tour, I had to use some words that are a mix of Scandinavian languages, so I wasn't using pure Norwegian.'

Feeling rather silly, Sue and I laughed. Then we chatted with her about how she came to be there and what she was doing. She was studying tourism and had been an exchange student in Longyearbyen in the past.

The bus soon went down along the water's edge and past a sign that read '*Velkommen til Longyearbyen havn | Bykaia*.'

It was welcoming us to the port of Longyearbyen, I thought.

Then I saw a red, black and white ship behind the sign. It was our ship, moored and waiting for us, with the large letters *Fram* brightly lit. On my maps, the port was south-west of the town of Longyearbyen, on a waterway, possibly a tiny fjord, off the end of a large fjord called Isfjord. The ship was moored alongside what looked like a parking and storage area just off the road.

I took a photo of the ship immediately. I wanted to create a starting place in my photo collection for the next part of our journey, but, more importantly, I was so excited to finally see the real thing. I'd only seen pictures of it before. The MS *Fram* was there before me, as I sat on the bus. A photo taken quickly, spontaneously, without too much setting up would capture my feelings and remind me of how excited I was before the cruise. (Photo 3.2.3)

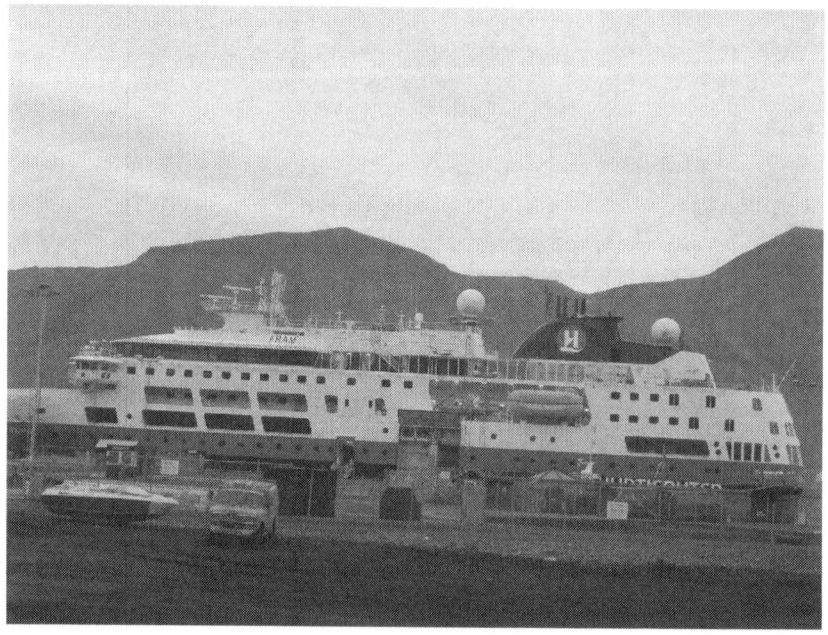

Photo 3.2.3 First sighting of the MS *Fram*

After we got off the bus and Sue and I had set up the scooter for the first time since the hotel, we all lined up and filed past a man at the entrance into a wire-fenced area around the ship. The small entrance served as a checkpoint before we were allowed to board.

After passing through, everyone went over to the ship. There was a short ramp going up from the bitumen base into one of the lower levels of the ship.

The whole bitumen area, which formed a wharf or pier, was only a small projection that extended out from the storage area. That was the meaning of another word on the sign that I saw earlier – *bykaia*. I looked it up later; it meant 'wharf'.

It was easy going up the ramp and inside the ship on my little yellow scooter. The ramp wasn't steep. I went into the entrance hall of Deck 3. My scooter and I and Sue were now on board the MS *Fram*.

I was keen to check out the ship as soon as possible. I wanted to see our room, the lounges, the dining room, the lecture rooms, everything. I particularly wanted to check that I could get around on my scooter without any help.

However, we had to line up again first. We had to register ourselves with our credit cards at a desk on Deck 3. There were two people working and I was surprised at how fast the two-hundred-odd passengers moved through the area.

As soon as we'd finished registration and put our ID tags around our necks, we took off. Sue and I walked and scootered just about everywhere. The lifts were great. They were big enough for me on my scooter, with room for at least four other people, and there were two of them. I checked the main dining room and there was a disabled toilet beside the other toilets.

Getting out on to the decks was a bit more difficult. There were short steep ramps with raised top ridges where two heavy doors closed together. One of the doors was in an open position and I could get up to the ridge and through, but it was difficult to turn the scooter after going straight up the ramp. I had to change direction; instead of going straight ahead, I had to turn a 90° angle. There wasn't enough room to turn with only one door open. My scooter was small and light but it was one metre long. I really needed someone to hold the other door open. Sue was usually with me but I did like to go off on my own at times to take a few photos.

There were two levels of decks to choose from. I tried both. Once outside on the decks, my scooter went well. I could really see what was all around me from out there. I could also ride the scooter to the rail and stand up for a while.

There was a wonderful panoramic observation lounge (Qilak Observation Lounge) on board, with tall glass windows and different levels in which to sit, relax and see outside. There were also two lecture rooms. That was where the scheduled lectures and presentations were going to be. It was all very nice, I thought.

In the cabin, the shower was the most important thing for me to look at first. The bathroom was immediately on the left of the cabin door as I entered. I saw that I'd be able to walk into the shower over a very small step and stand without any trouble. Fantastic, just what had been explained to me, I thought. The scooter fitted into the cabin too. It would need to be recharged every night, so that was good. The second most important thing was having a large window so I could see outside. That was there too. The whole ship was better than I'd ever thought it would be.

There was a lot of interesting information waiting on a small table in front of a comfy-looking chair. Our cruise ship, the MS *Fram*, was named after the polar ship *Fram*. That was the original ship that we'd seen in the Polarship Fram Museum in Oslo.

There was so much history behind the *Fram* – the history of polar exploration in the Arctic and Antarctic, and the role Norwegians had played in discoveries in both of those areas. The polar ship *Fram* went on several important expeditions in the late 1800s. There was Nansen's famous Arctic Ocean Drift, which went from 1893 to 1896. Nansen was trying to reach the North Pole. He took the *Fram* into the eastern Arctic Ocean and let her freeze into the pack ice. Then he waited for the ocean current drift to take her towards the pole. Nansen grew impatient after eighteen months. It was taking too long. He left the ship, taking a small team with dogs and sleds. He didn't reach the pole, but he did achieve the record of being the furthest person north at 86°13.6′N. But the story didn't end there.

While Nansen was sledding, the *Fram* continued to drift slowly westwards. She finally emerged into the North Atlantic Ocean on the natural east-west current of the Arctic Ocean, proving the current existed.

In a second expedition on the *Fram*, Nansen carried out scientific work and charted for the first time the west coast of Greenland and the northern Canadian islands. The *Fram* name was well worth having for our own ship.

Roald Amundsen, another Norwegian, was one of the most successful polar explorers of all time. He also used the polar ship *Fram*. He used it to get to and from Antarctica for his famous South Pole expedition. In December 1911, he was the first man to reach this destination, beating the Australians. I'd read about that too in the Polarship Fram Museum in Oslo.

Hurtigruten also provided information about their own MS *Fram*. They wrote:

Ship Description MS *Fram*
Year of construction – 2007
Ship Yard – Fincantieri, Italy
Passenger capacity – 318
Beds – 276
Car capacity – 0
Gross tonnage – 11,647
Length – 114 m
Beam – 20.2 m
Speed – 13 knots (24.08 km/h; 14.96 mph)

On their website, Hurtigruten said that 'MS *Fram* … designed for sailing in polar waters, holds the highest safety standards … the perfect size for optimum nautical manoeuvrability and guests' comfort.'

I found some more information later. I learned that the MS *Fram* had eight decks and an ice-class rating of 1B. It was registered in the port of Tromsø Norway and owned by the operator Hurtigruten.

Before leaving home, during the planning phase, I'd looked at the deck plan on the Hurtigruten website a number of times. Being on the ship in person and seeing it all, going to each of the eight decks, was more revealing and meant much more. After my exploration, I felt that I understood where things were and where I was at any moment. Most importantly, I could confidently get around on my yellow scooter without too many problems. Not only had my initial curiosity been satisfied but I also felt that I'd made a good choice with the MS *Fram*.

Sue had not looked too closely at the ship's details before we left but after our self-guided tour she said, 'You've done well. It's great.' I was pleased with myself.

I checked the time. Yes, the ship was about to depart at any minute. We waited, rugged up on deck, looking out at the mountains surrounding Longyearbyen. We'd seen a lot of the town and its surrounds that day. It all slipped away to our left as the ship moved out and away from the pier smoothly and gently. It was Cruise Day 1, Thursday 8 September, late in the afternoon. I felt content and I really hadn't given much thought to the next stop.

CHAPTER 3

THE SVALBARD: CRUISE PART 1

The MS *Fram* sailed south-west from Longyearbyen towards the sea, along Isfjord, the second-longest fjord in the Svalbard. But we didn't sail for long before we made our first stop at Barentsberg.

The port at Barentsberg was called our second landing and it was still Cruise Day 1. The expedition team called the time at Longyearbyen our first landing. They numbered the landings '1' and '2' for 8 September on a map that was placed on the notice-board later. (Photo 3.3.1)

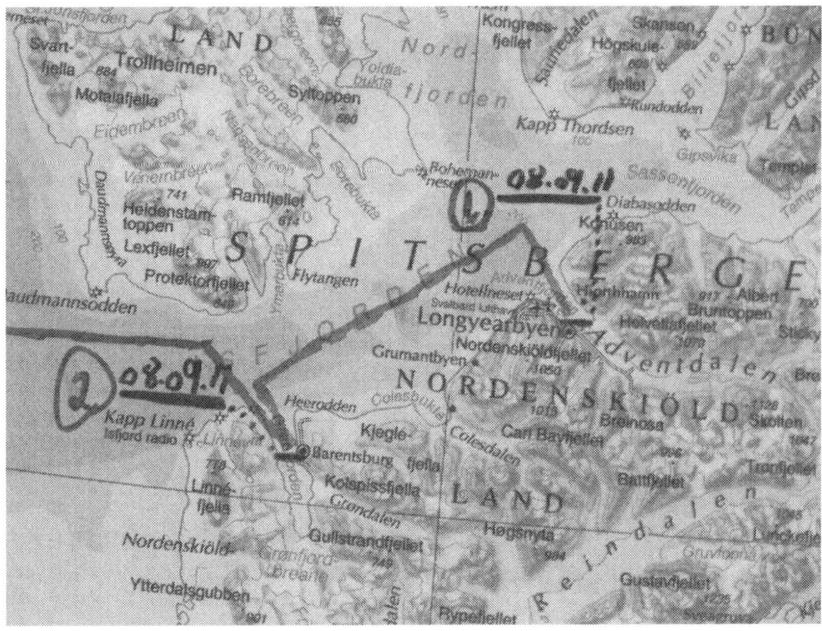

Photo 3.3.1 Map showing Svalbard, first and second landings

Barentsberg turned out to be only a short way away, once again in another smaller fjord off the larger Isfjord. Barentsberg is the site of a Russian settlement of about six hundred people, with an operating power station. They mine coal there, generate electricity and sell both on the open market.

The visit to Barentsberg was quite an event. The ship moored alongside soot-coated buildings of metal and concrete. For those going on foot, there were over two hundred steps to climb up a zigzag staircase. The staircase and a walkway rose up from the ground on piers and then went much higher up, disappearing among the buildings. I took a photo of a few hundred people climbing the stairs. This wooden staircase went up the side of the mountain as if it had grown out of it.

I disembarked on my scooter. A small 4WD bus, which looked like a military vehicle, was waiting to drive those of us who were unable to climb the stairs. Sue and I loaded the scooter on to it and I was able to step up and inside using a handrail. One of the supervisors said, 'I'd love to help, but according to O. H. & S rules, I can't. I'm not allowed. I don't have any care training.'

'That's fine, we'll manage,' I said, feeling quite surprised. The scooter didn't need to be lifted at once; it was just the front end that needed lifting first and then we rolled and pushed the back end in. It wasn't heavy if we moved it that way. I could lift up the front of the scooter and then lift myself up. Sue helped me lift my left leg a little at the end. There wasn't much training needed for that manoeuvre, I thought.

But, on thinking about it further, I realised that yes, someone really would have to know what we wanted done. They wouldn't know on their own. We'd have to tell them and they'd have to follow our instructions. The man's comment was fair enough. Besides, I'd become wary when people tried to help us because something could easily go wrong.

It was a bit of a rough ride up the steep, winding, narrow road to the settlement. When the dirt gravel road stopped, we got out on to coal-blackened slabs of concrete. There were slabs of varying sizes with gaps between them. Some gaps were up to thirty centimetres wide, others were much smaller. The slabs looked black and slimy, but my scooter went over them without any trouble. I picked the smallest gaps to go across.

We continued to climb up the mountainside, the walkers on the concrete slabs and me scootering along. We were going higher and higher and I wondered about the slope and getting back safely. It was nighttime and dark.

An enthusiastic Russian man was our guide. He told us about Barentsberg and the mining community. He spoke of its history and daily life. He talked on while taking us on winding paths, past living quarters and offices.

It looked to me like every picture I'd ever seen of communist Russia or East Berlin – barren. One wooden building lay at almost 45°, and looked like it was about to fall down. Painted in bright colours, it made a fantastic photograph. I scooted on and up, my mouth agape and my camera ready.

Images from Russian novels that I'd read in the 1970s sped across my mind. Alexander Solzhenitsyn is my favourite, and I had to keep his presence on my bookcase forever. Scenes from a movie about East Berlin, *The Lives of Others*, shunted in a ticker-tape line across my mind. I'd never been to East Berlin or Russia. Having it all in front of me was new, but also oddly old. It seemed sad and strange, like it belonged to the past. But it was still exciting for me to be there.

We went into a large wooden building that looked as if it served as a community hall. There was a small shop there, selling handicrafts such as knitted gloves, scarves and jumpers. There were also babushka dolls and odd trinkets that some people stopped to look at. But perhaps everyone was still in a bit of a daze after the Soviet visions outside.

We all moved forward into another large room, which turned out to be a theatre with an elevated stage at the front. The walls looked thin and colourless, and there were no decorations anywhere.

The locals had organised a five-person Russian dance show

with two musicians, all of whom worked at the mine. I rode my scooter to the row right at the front and sat in one of the seats.

A man and two women came on to the stage to sing and dance. Two male musicians played their instruments behind them at the rear of the stage. One of the instruments was an electric keyboard and the other looked like it might be a traditional Russian string instrument. They were all dressed in traditional Russian clothes.

The man playing the keyboard looked a bit like a transvestite, but I don't think he was. Maybe it was just his make-up. He had bright red lipstick on. It was all very bright in contrast to the surroundings, and we laughed and clapped along. The show was over in just under an hour. The whole thing was a total surprise to me.

We filed out and I started to think about the way back, down those steep slabs in the dark. But there was no need to worry. The military 4WD was outside the hall to take the non-walkers back to the ship. It had negotiated the paths up. After a bit of swaying and some raising of our eyebrows, we arrived back down at the bottom on to level ground beside the sea.

We boarded the ship using the ramp again, and swiped our name tags as we entered. The captain needed to know that all the passengers were back on board before sailing off. I didn't think anyone would choose to stay. Once on board, everyone went to the dining room for a late dinner.

After dinner, Sue and I went straight back to our cabin. It had been a long day, and we weren't even unpacked yet. We'd been in the same clothes all day. But everyone else had been dressed in the same casual way too. Sue unpacked our bag and hung some of our tops and pants up.

Sue was good in that way. She did the unpacking most of the time. Standing up to hang clothes was another slightly difficult task for me. There was usually nothing close by for me to lean on for support. Wardrobes and open hanging spaces aren't made that way. Sue said she was happy to do it so that was something else that she took charge of. It was a nice feeling, being cared for. 'What do you want to wear tomorrow? I'll put it out,' she'd say.

The ship sailed west and then south-west out of the fjords into the Norwegian and Greenland Seas. Then it headed north. It was dark and we couldn't see anything. Our television screen indicated our position on a map, while the video camera at the front of the ship showed the silent darkness around us. We went to bed and slept well.

By the next morning, Cruise Day 2, we had arrived in Magdalenefjord in the far north of the island of Spitsbergen. It's listed as a World Heritage Site for its stunning scenery.

I woke and looked through the window. Wow, glaciers! There were glaciers everywhere, five, six, more, it seemed. Each way I turned my head there was another glacier. The mountains were spiked and jagged.

We rose quickly, and showered and dressed for the day.

Our bathroom was very nice, I thought. I wasn't an expert on ship bathrooms, but it was certainly better for me than the one in the cabin on our last ship, the ship we took to Antarctica. Our bathroom on the MS *Fram* was much easier to move around in. The shower had a plastic sliding door and I could easily get in and out of it over a small step. The shower wasn't too big and it wasn't too small. I could lean, balance and hold on to things. The finishes were very nice too. This was the third ship I'd ever been on, but that bathroom was the best yet. I went on my first ship at the age of fifteen, when I was on my way back home from New Zealand with my family. I couldn't remember what the bathroom was like on that journey. It didn't mean much then.

Our third landing was in Magdalenefjord, at Grave Headland, or Gravneset. It was our first outing in the polar circle boats. We went in groups of ten. The expedition team organised the passengers into seven groups, and everyone had an allocated number and colour. We were in Group 4, red. There were announcements over the ship's public address system at various times for a particular number and colour to proceed to the disembarking deck, Deck 2.

When they announced our group, Sue and I went down. I went by the lift on my scooter and Sue used the stairs. When I arrived on Deck 2, I waited until the small crowd had cleared a bit before I started to organise myself. Sue gave me a life jacket and I waited for a clear entry to where the boots were.

A member of the crew came up to me and saw me sitting on my scooter. He said, 'Do you think you are going out over there, on to the rocks, snow and ice in that?'

'No,' I said. 'I just thought I'd use it to come down here to get my life jacket. I'll leave it in the corner over there out of the way for when I get back.' Of course I didn't think I was going to scooter over the snow, ice and rocks on the shore!

'I'll have to check with the expedition leader,' he said. He went away and came back in a few minutes. 'Yes, that's okay.'

I wasn't sure what he'd been checking but I'd continued preparing myself anyway. It'd never occurred to me that I couldn't go out on a polar circle boat. Not after I'd seen pictures of them, and not after having being on an inflatable Zodiac before.

Putting on a life jacket took a few go's. They were red and all piled on top of each other in a tall metal unit with two shelves. The metal unit was on wheels for easy moving in and out of the deck reception area just by the lifts.

The boots were in another room, called a muck room, off to the side of the disembarking area. All the boots were on a wooden rack and each single boot lived on a peg that projected out from the rack. They were grouped in twos. The pegs had cabin numbers written beside them.

The rubber gumboots were the most difficult things to get on. I wasn't the only one having trouble, either. A few people needed help with them. There was a special device on the floor that you could use to help get them off later. It held the boot while you pulled your foot and leg out of it. I thought I might try that when we came back.

Finally, I was fully dressed. I had a life jacket on over my waterproof top and pants, which were over a warm layer, which, in turn, was over thermal underwear. I was also wearing gloves and a beanie with earflaps. I was ready to go.

I stood in the line with Sue, using my walking stick. At the call, I moved outside past the crew member at the door. I swiped my ship ID card and name tag and went forward. After I'd walked a few metres, there was a set of stairs leading down to a platform on the water. There were handrails on either side of the stairs and there were about eighteen steps in all. I went down the steps slowly, one by one. There were people in front of me and people behind. Sue was immediately behind me, keeping watch.

Once down on the platform, with a crew member to lean on and a rail to grab, I stepped into the polar circle boat and sat on the long seat. The boat was soon full and a member of the team started the outboard motor. Off we went to shore. It was only a few hundred metres to a small, rocky, pebbly peninsula.

When we arrived, a team member on shore placed a set of portable metal steps in the shallow water at the top end of the boat. They were also there to offer a hand to help people move from the boat to shore. The handrail helped again too.

The rubber boots were most suitable for the few steps in the water to shore. But the ground was very rocky and it was a little difficult for me to walk on. I made it okay with an arm or two to lean on. I waited for Sue when I was out of the water, leaning on my walking stick. Sue helped me walk a few metres further to sit down on some flat rocks. I had a wonderful 360° view of at least four glaciers, snow-covered jagged mountains, the ship, the peninsula and the fjord. It was stunning.

I sat there and looked around in awe, soaking in the view. I had my camera tucked in my jacket, ready to use. When I looked through the viewfinder, I thought about what kind of scene I'd take. How could I possibly capture what was here and how I felt? There were too many choices! I took a lot of photos. I was trying to capture that one special scene that would remind me of how I felt being on the 'beach' of Gravneset in Magdalenefjord.

I'd expected to be able to travel in a polar circle boat. But I really didn't have much of an idea of what would come afterwards. I certainly didn't expect to be sitting on a beach by a fjord looking out at endless glaciers. I loved being there.

My favourite photo was the one I took of our expedition leader standing with a rifle over her shoulder. She was looking out across the water and watching three polar bears. (Photo 3.3.2)

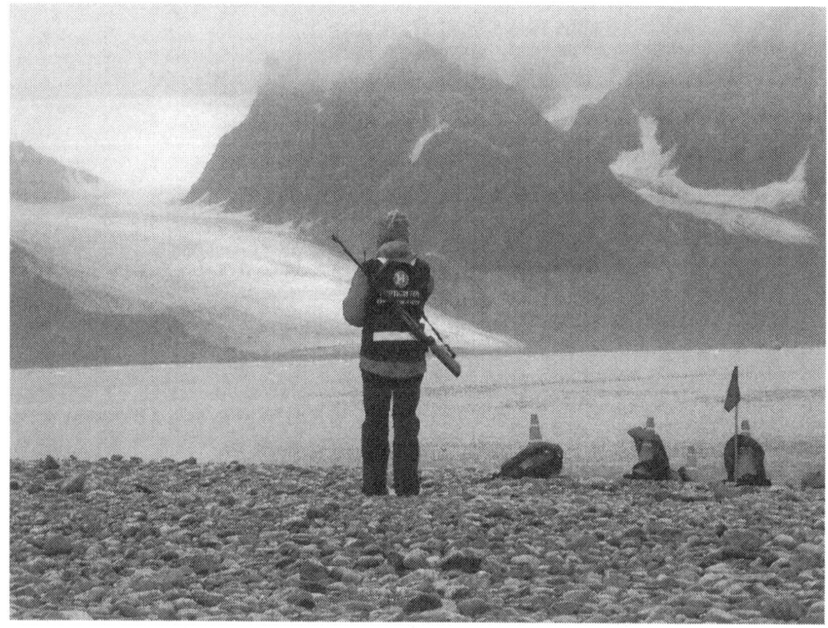

Photo 3.3.2 My favourite photo – Magdalenefjord

Our expedition leader had warned us that there were polar bears across the bay. If they went into the water and started swimming, she'd announce an immediate evacuation back to the boat. There would be 'little time to waste. The bears are fast swimmers,' she said.

Meanwhile, everyone else went on a walk towards a deserted-looking hut on my right, near the base of a mountain. There was also to be a long walk to Gully Glacier and a shorter walk to a whaler graveyard, where there were the remains of blubber ovens used during the whaling period of 1600 to 1700. The cemetery contained about a hundred and thirty graves in a fenced-off area. Sue went on the shorter walk. The uneven pebbled surface would have made for slow-going on the long walk, with her bad knee.

In those icy waters of Magdalenefjord, we had the option of taking a 'polar plunge'. The expedition team had brought towels ashore just in case. Anyone who tried it would get a special certificate for braving the waters. But I didn't see anyone swimming while I was sitting there. As for me, I love swimming, but not in icy-cold water!

When Sue came back, she was with Glenda. Glenda was in her eighties and had a walking-stick seat with her. I thought Glenda had done well to walk over such an uneven surface. I was sitting on the pebbles with my legs stretched out by then. I couldn't get up. Sue offered me an arm but I felt I needed more than that. I needed to turn myself around somehow, to lean on something and push myself up. I was getting a bit worried and, as I was trying to figure it out, Glenda said, 'Here, use this. I find I have the same trouble.' She unfolded her seat and put it beside me. I leant on it and it did make it much easier. I felt better.

'Oh, thank you, Glenda,' I said. 'That really helped.' I thought I must remember that kind of seat for myself for another time.

It was time to leave. We walked the short distance to our pile of life jackets at the edge of the shore and each of us put one on. When the next boat came to shore, we stepped up and in, and were soon motoring back to the ship. Once we were at the platform on the side of the ship, I stepped out with help from the crew and ascended the stairs one by one. That was my first wet landing.

Once inside the ship again, on Deck 2, we took off our life jackets and went into the muck room to take off our rubber boots. I tried to use that device to help me take off my boots, but I gave up. I had to get Sue to help me pull them off. We put the boots back on to the pegs over our cabin number.

We'd had to hire the boots. We'd gone for fittings soon after we'd boarded the day before. They were all new. We'd rented them for the twelve days on the ship, but that was the only time I wore them. Sue had one more wet landing, so she wore her boots twice.

When most people seemed to be back on board the ship, there was an announcement. There was going to be a delay in our departure. A man had fallen and broken some bones. A medical retrieval helicopter was coming to land on the small peninsula to take him to hospital. The ship couldn't leave until that had happened. The place was beautiful enough just to sit and look at for a lot longer anyway. Waiting was no problem

An emergency evacuation safety drill was also scheduled for that time. As instructed, we noted our assembly station, which was written in the safety instructions on the inside of our cabin door. There was an announcement over the PA system and we all followed the instructions given. We went to our station out on the deck and watched a crew member demonstrate how to put on a large orange flotation suit. He looked quite odd. There was a lot of laughter mixed with the seriousness of the demonstration. I hoped we wouldn't end up in the water. My scooter would definitely not fit in the suit!

Then another announcement – three polar bears (the ones across the bay) were still there, on cliffs near a glacier. The ship sailed closer and everyone came out on deck. I set up my camera on the railing to steady it. The polar bears were a long way away on some sparse green vegetation between the rocks. They were just moving white blobs. I zoomed in and took as many photos as I could while trying to hold the camera steady.

Some of the photos I took were at a focal length (in 35-millimetre film equivalent) of 678, 1,763 and 2,441 millimetres. With such a large superzoom, the photos were all slightly blurry, but at least I'd seen the polar bears and captured them. I knew I went well over the optical zoom range into the digital zoom range. There was a lot of excitement on board – they were the first polar bears we'd seen on the trip.

Before we left, Gwen had said, 'You probably won't see too many polar bears because you'll be on the warmer, western side of Spitsbergen. The ship I was on was a polar vessel – an icebreaker – and we went around to the other, colder, eastern side. That's where most of the polar bears are. There's more snow and ice there.'

'Oh, I hope we see at least some,' I'd said. 'I think we will.' I'd wanted to think that we would. I'd needed to. And here they were!

We watched the bears walk over the rocks looking for food. They were thin, and it seemed a bit sad. I saw only two of them, both adults. As I could later see on my enlarged photos, their noses were longer than I'd imagined. Their paws were big and wide, and their ears were little and cute. They did look very cuddly, but I'm sure they weren't interested in a cuddle. It was food that they were after. The ship drifted slowly past the bears and they disappeared from our sight.

People were rushing about with their cameras, very excited with their photos, saying to each other, 'Oh, look at this!', 'Wow, what did you take that on? What were the settings?', 'Show me yours, please,' and 'You should see Joe's over there.'

There was a mix of languages but the excitement was clear. Although my photos were a bit blurry, they were among the closest that I saw. But Gwen's were much, much better. And clearer. Not blurry at all.

A couple of hours after the announcement about the injured passenger, we heard helicopter blades whirring overhead. As unfortunate as it was for the man himself, everyone was keen to see the action so they positioned themselves to get a good view. That included me.

The helicopter landed on the pebbly shore. Two uniformed paramedics got out with a stretcher and went over to the group of people looking after the man. They carried him to the helicopter and flew away. There was another announcement to let us know what was happening. They'd keep us informed of how the man got on, and the ship would now depart Magdalenefjord.

It was late in the afternoon, and, by the time the ship finally left, I was in our cabin having a rest. We moved west out of the fjord towards the sea. I got up and went back upstairs to look at what was passing by. We sailed through Smeerenburgfjord, another beautiful area. The icy mountains and glaciers slid by. Once we were out at sea, we headed north again, to Moffen Island.

Not far from Moffen Island, there was another announcement.

We saw a herd of walruses lying on a large area of raised black sand in the ocean, like a tidal island. There were about thirty or fifty of them. Most were huddled close together, almost on top of each other. The ship wasn't allowed to get too close. We had to keep a prescribed distance of three hundred metres between them and us. There were rules in the Arctic about protecting animals in their native habitat.

Through my superzoom telephoto lens, I could see the tusks on the male bulls and the babies feeding from their mothers. With my naked eye, the walruses just looked like grey blobs. I looked at the properties information for one of my photos and saw that I'd taken that photo at a digital focal length of 192 millimetres and that focal length in 35-millimetre film was 1,085. That was still enormous, I thought, but not quite so blurry. I felt great being able to see the walruses in their natural environment. I think I could smell them too!

A little later, when we arrived within view of Moffen Island, there was yet another announcement. 'Welcome to the furthest point north that we will sail. Please join us in a celebration drink that the crew will now serve on the deck.'

They served schnapps in plastic glasses. I put ours on the ship's outer rail ledge, with the ocean and island behind, to take a photo. Then I took a photo of Glenda with Sue, clinking glasses to mark the event. The sun was starting to set and the sky was pink. It was lovely.

Soon after that, the team delivered certificates to our cabin. They all had our names on them. Mine read:

ARCTIC CERTIFICATE
Maureen Corrigan
Aboard MS *Fram*
Reached the Northern Latitude of
N 80°00′ E 14° 27′
On the 9th of September 2011 at 21:50 Hrs

It was a significant achievement. I felt chuffed that I'd been able to get that far north and into the Arctic. We were almost at the North Pole!

When I got back to the cabin shortly afterwards, our bearings and location were showing on the television screen. I took a photo to record our achievement and where we were. (Photo 3.3.3)

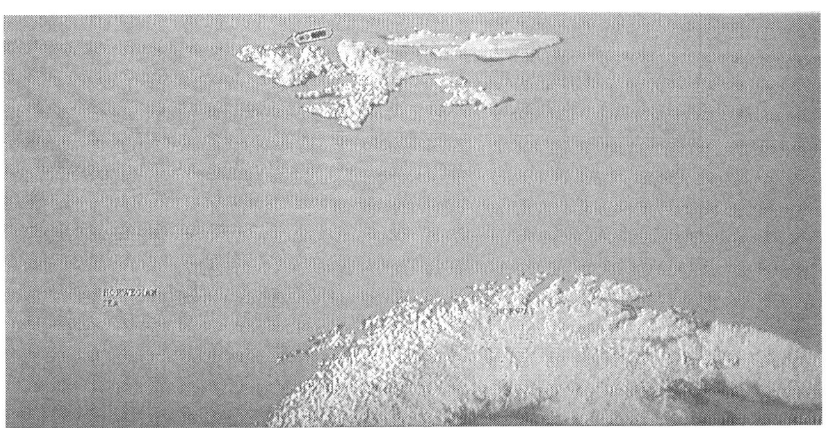

Photo 3.3.3 Map of ship's location near Moffen Island

I looked at our position again. We really were a long way north in the world, right at the very top.

Overnight, the ship turned and went back south, a long way west of Spitsbergen. We travelled past the latitude of Magdalenefjord and went further south before turning east towards the coast again. We arrived at our fourth landing of Ny-Ålesund on the morning of Cruise Day 3. We were once again on Spitsbergen, north of Longyearbyen.

The ship moored at a pier almost in the middle of a little village. We were at the northernmost inhabited point in the world, a research station. Several nations had an interest in this place in the Svalbard. From onboard the ship, I could read a noticeboard that said:

Welcome to Ny-Ålesund

A strong and attractive international Arctic research community

...centre for Arctic environmental monitoring and research...

.... dependent on a near-pristine environment, therefore some special rules apply...

The rules were listed. Stay on the marked roads and don't touch anything summed them up, I think.

Also on display was the weather forecast for the next nine days. The temperatures read 5°, 3°, 3°, 1°, 0°, -1°, 0°, 1° and 3°C.

There was an announcement on the ship's PR system the night before we arrived telling us that the most northern post office in the world was in this village. To have a postcard sent from there would be special, we thought. Sue and I wrote at least six postcards.

Sue disembarked and went for a walk with a small group around the village of Ny-Ålesund and posted the postcards on that day, 10 September.

I stayed on the ship. I could see that the dirt road was muddy and wet and it was raining a little on and off. I didn't want to take my scooter out on to the muddy surface, even though it was flat. It might be slippery and the mud might affect the electric motor, I thought. We were only up to Day 10 of our trip; there was much more ahead of us yet.

I sat in the observation lounge on a nice comfy chair, looking out at the town and the whiteness surrounding it. I read about the settlement. There was a small but good library in the lounge.

Roald Amundsen started his expeditions to the North Pole from Ny-Ålesund. His first attempts were by seaplane, but they weren't successful. Then, in 1926, he left Ny-Ålesund in a giant Zeppelin and flew over the North Pole and Alaska, and back again.

How interesting, I thought, and went on to think that I might have seen a Zeppelin in some documentaries about early air travel. I knew experiments in flying became a reality in the late 1800s and early 1900s. Zeppelin airships looked very different to the other craft being trialled at that time. They were large rigid structures filled with bags of hydrogen gas and driven by engines. They were a little like those blimps that fly over sporting events, but blimps are much smaller and more like elongated balloons. Air travel has certainly come a long way since then. Those early polar explorers must have been very brave to fly at that time.

I put on my blue wind jacket and went out on deck to look at the village and its surrounds more closely. I imagined a giant Zeppelin flying out over the land and the water to get to the North Pole.

There was a lot of water to the north of the Svalbard. I love the explanation I read once about the difference between the North and South Poles – the North Pole was in water surrounded by land and the South Pole was on land surrounded by water. That summed it up quite well, I thought.

Looking at the streets of Ny-Ålesund, I could see a lot of blue jackets walking about. Everyone on board our ship had a blue wind jacket. On the first day, after we'd boarded and registered, we went straight to a room full of jackets. We'd given Hurtigruten our sizes months before. The jackets were all the same wonderful bright sky-blue colour. I really liked them. We were allowed to keep them after the trip. The blue reminded me of the bright blue Australian sky, especially at Broome. We were a long way from Broome!

The bright blue of the jackets really stood out against the snow, the ice and the pale blue skies of the Svalbard. The expedition team wore red. On our earlier Antarctic trip, we'd had red jackets and the expedition team had had yellow. I could see that, either way, with those colours, it was easy to spot people from a cruise whenever they were off the ship, wherever they were.

When Sue came back from her walk, I was lost in my thoughts but she was keen to talk. 'You won't believe it but as I was looking at some figures of Chinese lions outside a building, I happened to look ahead and saw a group of blue wind jackets wandering off together past the sign that read "Do Not Proceed Past this Point, Danger of Bears".'

The expedition team had warned us about the polar bears

many times. They'd also said that at this particular landing, several members of the expedition team would go ahead and check if it was safe for us to disembark. I saw them head off with rifles over their shoulders shortly after we moored.

Sue continued. 'I could see and read the sign with a wave of blue disappearing behind it into the distance. There were two choices for a walk when I got out there. You could either go with a guide or go on your own. I went on my own, but I didn't follow them past the sign.'

'What happened then?' I asked.

'Nothing. I just went off on my own and saw where Amundsen had taken off, in some sort of giant balloon I think.'

'But what about the group of people going beyond the sign?' I asked.

'I didn't see or hear any bears. So they must have come back okay. It was a bit risky, though.'

Expecting a more dramatic ending to the story, I wasn't sure what to say. 'Oh, okay,' I said. Then I thought they must have had a guide with a rifle somewhere among them. There were no PR announcements before the ship departed, so everything must have been in order. Sue must have just been amazed that people would do that.

'Did you post the postcards?' I asked.

'Yes,' said Sue. 'The postbox was just a red metal box with a hole in it.'

I'll always remember the date that Sue posted the postcards because it was eight months later that they finally started arriving! 'Thanks for your postcard,' Our friend Brenda said when she rang to let us know in 2012. 'I didn't think you'd left on this year's holiday yet. Then I read the date on the card. It says "9 September 2011" but the postmark reads "13 May 2012". Oh dear, that's taken a long time!'

Eventually, we learned that only five of the six postcards posted at Ny-Ålesund actually arrived. I received an SMS message from Carolyn the year after we returned, sometime in 2012, which said

'Our PO Box has just given birth to a beautiful PC called Longyearbyen conceived on 9/9/11. Thank you…'

I found out much later that the postcards left Ny-Ålesund the following year when the winter ice had melted, allowing a ship in to pick up the mail. I didn't think at the time how the postcards would leave the settlement.

When our ship was ready to leave, about ten people from the Ny-Ålesund community came out to give us a special farewell. They formed a marching band and played a trumpet, a trombone and drums. They carried a banner which said, 'Ny-Ålesund Slag & Blase Ensemble 79°N'. There was also a sign that said something like 'Farewell to the last ship to visit us this year'. Even then, it didn't occur to me what being on the last ship to call in at Ny-Ålesund in 2011 meant for our postcards!

In the bistro area of the ship, on Deck 4, the expedition team had put up marked maps for us to see where we'd been. I took a photo of the route and the stops they'd drawn among the islands in the north-west and north of the Svalbard after we left Barentsberg. (Photo 3.3.4)

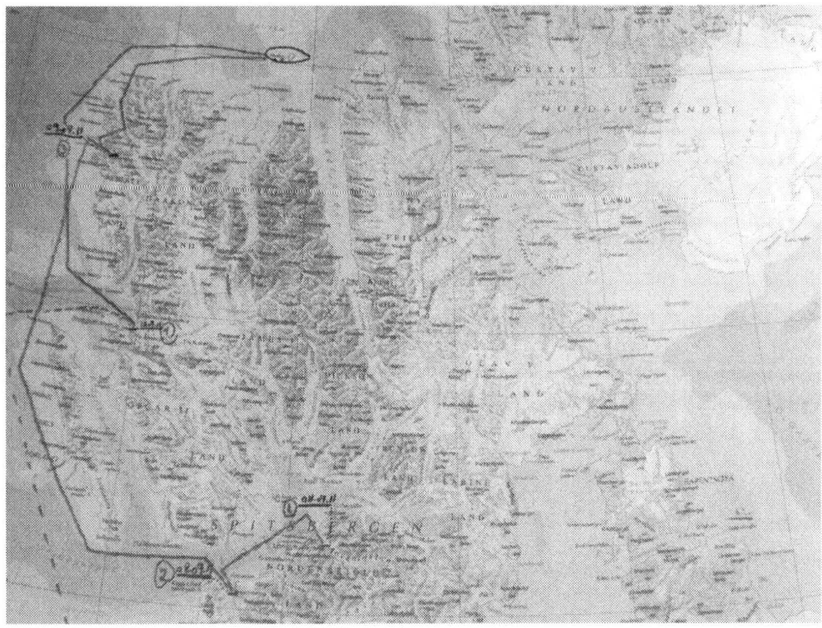

Photo 3.3.4 Map of our route north-west and north of the Svalbard to Moffen Island

From Ny-Ålesund, we headed west out to sea again. I kept an eye out for polar bears on the land and islands we passed. I'd been looking out ever since I saw the first two. Once or twice, I thought I could see a white speck moving in the distance. But, in the end, we didn't see any more polar bears in the Svalbard. Gwen was right. But at least we saw two of the three spotted at Magdalenefjord and they were in the wild.

There were no icebergs about either, just small craggy bits of ice in the water. The icebergs we'd seen in Antarctica were huge, the size of houses or football fields, and sometimes they were kilometres long. The larger icebergs of the northern hemisphere must, like the bears, be in a different region.

We left the Svalbard and headed south to cross the Norwegian Sea and the North Sea between Spitsbergen and mainland Norway. We had two full days at sea ahead of us, with one stop to come at Bear Island. We were still well above the Arctic Circle and would stay above it for many more days yet.

Lectures and talks on the ship were held in two rooms near the bistro. There were naturalists, geologists, scientists and other experts on board the ship to give talks and lead walks. In Paghøga Hall, the talks were mostly in German, while talks in the Framheim Hall were in English. While we were at sea on those two days, the expedition team scheduled even more talks for us than usual. I enjoyed listening to all of them and learned a lot about that area of the world.

It was during those two days that we met Thilli and Anni, who were from Germany. Thilli spoke some English, but seemed a little rusty. My Australian accent probably didn't help and I think I also spoke too fast. Thilli had learned English in London. Anni spoke just about no English at all – much like me with German. However, we all seemed to communicate and get along well. We had several meals together and started to get to know each other. We also met out on deck a few times, and continued to chat and share time together as the trip progressed.

I also came to know a few other people, such as Bruce. When we were staying at the hotel in Longyearbyen, I noticed a man walking with two tall walking sticks or poles. They had peculiar rubber feet on them. When I spoke with him at dinner one night, he told me that he had neuropathy. 'Doctors don't know the cause of it,' he said. 'They don't know the treatment for it, either. I have trouble feeling my feet.'

'Have you seen a neurologist?'

'Yes, I've seen a lot of specialists, and had many tests and scans. There's no definite answer.'

He walked with a slow shuffle. But he could cover quite long distances, I noticed.

We sat with Bruce and his wife Helen for a few meals. They were from Colorado in the USA. After a short time, Helen said she felt as if we were family. We felt comfortable chatting to each other and words soon slipped out more easily. I noticed that Bruce would often go off on his own; he'd look around and then stop, thinking quietly. I could identify with him. I had some good talks with Bruce

All our meals were served in the Imaq Restaurant on Deck 4. Food and meals were that great human necessity and social occasion. 'You are what you eat' I hear, and that makes me think about healthy eating, food, life and death.

***

I don't very often think about what might happen to me in the end – or near the end, or, in fact, quite possibly well before the end. But, occasionally, the thought might flash past. It's become something to consider ever since I was diagnosed with MS. I sometimes heard about what had happened to other people with MS. Images of young people bedridden in nursing homes were probably the worst. I'm very lucky. Lucky so far, and maybe I will be right until the end. There's a lot more time ahead yet, I hope. There are also a lot of things I can still control.

Since my diagnosis, I've paid even greater attention to what I eat and how I exercise. I don't want to one day be sitting in a bariatric wheelchair if I can help it. It's hard enough walking at my normal weight. If I were heavier, it would be even harder.

I read the magazines and newsletters that the MS societies publish. They have good advice in them and usually include news about some of the latest research. I read in one of them about a study that seemed to indicate a link between high blood-fat levels, levels of disability and rates of disability progression. It seems that simple lifestyle choices such as diet and exercise might slow the rate of progression by lowering the level of bad saturated fats circulating in the body. I'm keen to do whatever I can to help slow my MS progression. So I took extra note.

I'm a big fan of Doctor Rosemary Stanton, who has a PhD in nutrition. I love reading her articles, which always acknowledge proper published scientific research. Her ideas always make such great common sense to me, and she knows her facts. I also love that her advice always ends up with the same answer – that we need a good, balanced diet with less saturated fat, less sugar and more fruit, vegetables, legumes and whole grains.

I've tried to eat healthy food for a very long time, even before I finished studying medicine. An entry in my senior yearbook from 1977 makes mention of it – '...her health food diet and obvious physical fitness...' I probably even said 'You are what you eat' back then, proselytising while I smoked! (I did eventually give up.)

University days in the 1970s in Sydney were fantastic for a sort-of country girl like me. A hundred kilometres was a long way away from the exciting restaurants in Australia's biggest city. I was part of a group of friends who called ourselves the 'Gourmet Gobblers'. We went out every few months to a different restaurant. I loved experiencing all those new foreign foods and wines. It seemed so exotic. Those were the days, as they say!

I do still like going out to some of the best restaurants now and then. I've been around Australia with the Australian Gourmet Traveller Restaurant Guide packed in my bag. So I like nice food.

Nice, fresh, healthy, terrific-tasting food! If I eat a fatty meal, my body doesn't like it and I feel different afterwards. I like feeling healthy and I want to maintain that feeling every day.

I'm proud that I've always weighed about the same, ever since my early twenties. I've remained a size 12 too. But I do have to work at it. I can't do the same sort of exercise these days as I used to, so I have to watch what I eat.

Diet, with its obvious connection to health and weight, seems to have become a very difficult issue for many people and for so many different reasons. It can be a taboo subject.

There also seems to be so much incorrect information everywhere, trying to con people into a quick fix or a pill rather than what is needed – a slower and more difficult change in lifestyle. I was a GP; I looked after people for ten years and thought I did a good job most of the time. But I'm sure I wasn't very good at helping people lose weight. I was too blunt and matter of fact – 'Oh, and don't have chips, soft drinks or lollies'. This advice was correct but my direct approach wasn't the most helpful.

Eating seems to have become a social problem in our affluent Western world, with levels of obesity and related illnesses rising all the time. I was a doctor and cared. That's why I did medicine, to try and help people. And relying on evidence and science rather than opinions was in my make-up. But I came to realise that fixing the problem in my part of the world was not as simple as I thought it was. I like fixing things but I can't fix that for anyone else. I can, however, give it a go for myself.

I also know that I'm very lucky and privileged to be in my current position in life, to have a choice and to know something about what to choose. 'Luck' has a lot to do with everything, I've come to realise. There are three main causative factors in illness – genes, lifestyle and luck. For some people, no matter how hard they try to live a healthy lifestyle, if genes and luck aren't in their favour then the odds are really stacked against them. No one can control that.

With regards to lifestyle, there is a choice, and most people are free to choose what they want. People can make all sorts of choices.

Some people even elect not to have any treatment for an illness. That's their choice and their right, and I have mine too.

I've been to one or two philosophical talks and discussions. It's interesting to think a bit about beliefs, values, attitudes and other aspects of life from time to time. But as with languages and being artistic, I'm not very talented in the philosophy department.

Choice, and the freedom to choose, are some of the most important things about living, along with good luck. Being independent is part of that too. I'm still able to make choices about my life.

But what would I do if I couldn't make certain choices any more? What if I couldn't control my electric wheelchair and take myself where I wanted to go? What if I couldn't do anything very much any more? What if I become bedridden?

I did a Myers-Briggs Type Indicator test when I was still working. It turns out that I like to be prepared well ahead of time and not leave things to the last minute. I have a will and have made my end-of-life choices known. I've organised all the recommended legal documents.

I also like to think that I'd react to a big change in my health by thinking 'Well, I'll just have to deal with it'.

In the meantime, I'm just going to get on with enjoying life, every day and every meal.

***

It was time for lunch and fortunately there was much to choose from on the MS *Fram*.

The Imaq Restaurant was towards the aft (the rear) of the ship. The lifts to get there were in the middle of the ship on Deck 4. After I rode out of the lift, I'd go into a lobby with windows from floor to ceiling. Then I'd go down a wide hallway, with more windows to look out of. To my right, leading to the restaurant, there were toilets. There was a great disabled toilet just near the others, and it was clearly signposted. These days, I noticed where the toilets were like I'd never noticed them before! Toilets and power points – they were just little things but they'd become so important in my life now.

I reverse-parked my scooter just up from the disabled toilet. I left it against the wall, out of the way and only a few steps away from the restaurant. That was a great parking spot, I thought.

Sue waited so I could hold her arm and walk in using my walking stick. At the entrance, we used the hand sanitiser, which had a big sign by it asking everyone to please use it. Once inside, we stood and scanned the tables and people to decide where we'd sit. There were usually plenty of spots available. Luckily, there was open seating at all meal times so we could choose where we wanted to sit. I'd heard of other cruises with set places and no choice. I wouldn't have liked that.

A buffet of food was arranged in the centre with tables surrounding the displays and grouped in a C-shape. The food on the ship was good. There were great choices at every meal. In particular, there were healthy options – plenty of fresh fruit and vegetables.

Once we'd found seats, I'd sit down straight away. Sue would go off and get some food for both of us. Sue knew what I liked and what was good for me. She took particular care of what I ate.

I thought she had a vested interest. A few times, when we'd been at an airport and I had to check the scooter in with the baggage, Sue was left to push me in a wheelchair. Airport wheelchairs are never light, smooth or fast. Sue might have said at least once, 'I'm glad you're not fat, it's hard enough as it is,' or 'The wheels just won't go properly on this wheelchair… Imagine if you were bigger.'

At breakfast, Sue made a great cereal mix at the buffet, put natural yoghurt on it and brought over lots of fruit to go with it. I'd bring my psyllium husks to the table and religiously add two dessertspoons to my food every morning. At least one of my friends had called my favourite type of breakfast 'chaff', but it tasted good to me. The brewed coffee wasn't terrific but we managed.

At lunchtime, Sue often said, 'There's so many different salad vegetables to choose from,' and she brought lots of different kinds with different colours arranged beautifully on the plate. To add to the salad, there was a good variety of fish, meats and cheeses to choose from. The bread was good too, eaten with 'no fat' as Sue would say – that is, no margarine or butter. Those spreads were cultural habits I'd lost some time ago; that was Sue's influence. She was famous for it. If moisture was required, I used avocado or extra virgin olive oil.

But Sue did have a vice. She said that if she was going to eat fat (or had to), then she'd make sure it was good quality! She liked the best 'real' butter, ice cream and chocolate.

Dinner at night was mostly a buffet too and sometimes it was a set three-course menu. For the set menus, they took orders the day before, with a few alternatives. There were two sittings for set dinners, one early and one late, depending on which group you were in.

Sometimes, at the end of a day, my left hand would feel weak and I found it hard to turn my wrist and hold a fork to cut something. I had to ask Sue for help. I found it embarrassing, but Sue understood and no one seemed to notice her cutting my meat. I used the fork in my right hand to eat. Bad table manners, according to what I was taught, but I couldn't help it.

There was always a large selection of traditional desserts too – cakes, pastries and puddings. I noticed that the queue was always crowded in that section of the buffet! Sue and I both rarely ate those kinds of desserts. We usually had some fresh fruit instead. And there was some lovely fruit there. But, sometimes, dessert was just too tempting. Not the big yucky cakes, but perhaps a lemon tart, a flavoured ice cream, a crumble or a pavlova (for Sue – yes!). They were things that we did sometimes eat and did enjoy. But in moderation, of course!

The wine at dinner wasn't too bad, either. There was a choice of a labelled bottle or the house white or house red by the glass. We tried both the labelled and the house in the beginning. The house won out; its quality was okay. Then we discovered that the house came in a bottle too, not just by the glass or small carafe. And, the most important thing about that was we could put the cork back in after we'd had what we wanted, and the waiter would write our room number on the bottle for the next night. We could make one bottle last two nights for two people. It was cheaper that way and controlled our intake nicely as well. That is, except when one or both of us wanted a white as well as a red! Then there were two corked and labelled bottles for a few more days. They held up surprisingly well even though they weren't supposed to last that long.

Late in the afternoon of Cruise Day 4, we sailed near Bear Island. It was windy and wet. The ship moored a fair way out from the island. It was alone in the middle of nowhere, about halfway between Spitsbergen, which was 220 kilometres away, and the coast of Norway.

Bear Island is the southernmost island of the Svalbard. When it was discovered in 1596, by the Dutch Arctic explorer Willem Barentsz, a polar bear was killed there, hence its name. The island is about twenty kilometres long, with vertical cliffs rising steeply out of the ocean all around it.

An announcement told us that there was a beach on the island with a rough path leading up to a plateau of lakes. Members of our expedition team were going to the island to see if conditions were suitable for a landing that afternoon.

They went out in the polar circle boats. I watched them disappear between two large rocks in the distance and turn left. After about ten minutes, they came back. There was another announcement that called for Group Numbers 7, 6, 5 and 4 to assemble on Deck 2 in the lobby. The announcement also said that after twenty to thirty minutes, they'd be calling Group Numbers 3, 2 and 1. They said it was going to be another wet landing and recommended that people wear rubber boots or waterproof Gore-Tex shoes.

Despite the rain and wind, many people ventured out. That was our fifth landing. I decided not to go. I watched from the warm, dry observation lounge, with its wonderful big windows.

Sue went out and I tried to take a photo of her in the polar circle boat, but it was a bit rough out there and the rain was coming directly at me on to the window. So my photo was a mess!

I learned from reading the ship's notes that there'd been some small-scale coal-mining work on the island for about seven years from 1918 until 1925. Its real claim to fame is that it is home to one of the largest sea bird colonies in the North Atlantic. Large populations of birds come to breed there. Surprisingly, there are also Arctic foxes in summer and polar bears in winter. The bears arrive there on drift ice. Amazing, I thought. Imagine looking out and seeing an iceberg go by with a polar bear on it. That would be something extra-special.

Oh, it looked so miserable outside! I was pleased that I'd decided not to go. The clouds hung low and the rocky outcrops were black and jagged. Apparently, the highest peak on the island was called Misery Mountain.

Sue returned, wet but happy. They'd landed on the beach and walked to the top of the island. Sue had met a woman named Kerrie on the walk and they came back with some fabulous photos of tiny Arctic flowers that they'd seen on the plateau.

Kerrie was one of the other two Australians on the trip. Kerrie and her husband Bob came from the Gold Coast in Queensland. Bob didn't go out either. The little flowers in the photos looked beautiful, with so many different colours. I thought they were lovely and I was really surprised that they grew there.

After a hot shower and a change of clothes, Sue was ready for dinner and a glass of wine. I went back to our cabin with her and took a photo of our location as shown on the television screen. (Photo 3.3.5)

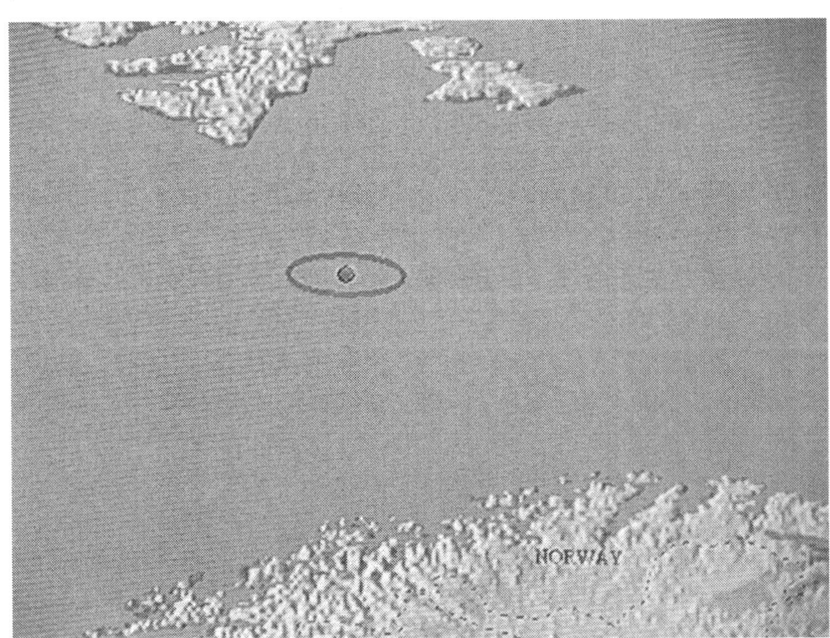

Photo 3.3.5 Map showing Bear Island

Sue told me more about the climb up the hill from the beach and about walking over lichen and moss with little flowers just everywhere. Sue and Kerrie had talked about the four of us meeting for dinner that night.

So we joined Kerrie and Bob for dinner. We were the only four Australians on the ship and had matching accents. 'Have you been on this ship before?' Bob asked.

'No,' I said. 'This is the first time. But I've been looking at where else this ship goes. I noticed it goes down to the Antarctic in a few months' time.'

'We're going on another Hurtigruten cruise on this ship, straight after this one finishes,' said Bob.

'Oh really? Where does that one go?'

'Well, after it leaves Bergen, the cruise goes up to the Orkney Islands off Scotland. Then it sails out to other remote islands off the coast of Ireland.'

'Wow, that sounds really interesting,' I said.

'We usually go off on our own sailing trips,' said Kerrie. 'It's new for us to be on an organised cruise.'

'Does that mean you have your own boat?' asked Sue.

'Yes. It's only small, but we've done a few trips on it,' said Bob. 'Now that we're retired, we can get away more often. It's a bit hard to bring it up here, though. So we booked this trip with Hurtigruten to travel north of Scotland and over to Ireland.'

'I'm not sure how we're going to go with it. I think I'll know better about what to expect another time, after this trip,' added Kerrie.

'How long have you had MS?' asked Bob.

'I was sort of diagnosed in 2001, so that's ten years. But I wasn't really diagnosed properly until 2006. And then I learned that I'd probably had it for much longer than that. It was all a bit confusing in the beginning.'

'That's interesting.'

'In the end, my neurologist thought that my first episode might have been in 1991, when I had some pain in my left arm and hand, coming from my neck. After a few months, I recovered completely from that, apart from odd numb sensations in my left hand. So that's twenty years ago.'

'You've done well,' said Bob.

'Yes, and for ten years I didn't know I might have MS. I had no symptoms at all. Just those funny numb feelings in my hand every now and then that never went away.'

***

Those symptoms in my left hand, arm and neck started after I did some building work. I used to enjoy being a handywoman sometimes. For hours, I'd been pressing down and turning a screw, using a screwdriver in my right hand. I was building a shed on the farm where I lived. I was determined to finish it by the end of the weekend.

The pain down my left arm and in my left hand started the next day and it didn't go away. I had a CT scan of my cervical spine during the weeks that followed. That was in 1991 and I was in my late thirties. The scan showed narrowing of some of the disc spaces. I saw a neurologist and he thought my symptoms were probably the result of pressure on some of the nerves in my cervical spine. He said that with time any nerve injury should recover. He told me the number of centimetres a nerve should repair and regrow each month. It would only take a few months.

I counted the months for a while and the pain did settle. But the funny tingly feelings in my left hand remained and have never stopped recurring for twenty years.

My current neurologist thinks it could have been an episode of brachalgia. Brachalgia is severe pain from a problem involving the brachial nerves in the cervical spine. There were many causes of this complaint, but he thinks it might have been my first episode of MS.

MRI scans were not around then. If they had been, my life would have been very different, I'm sure. After that arm and hand episode, I just continued living as I had been, thinking nothing had changed.

***

Bob was saying, 'Yes, they say diagnosing MS is difficult sometimes, don't they?'

'Yes, although MRIs are pretty good at picking up the lesions. But that alone isn't enough to say it's MS. It's funny, even though I did have my first MRI in 2001, my neurologist at the time said it was just a bit of inflammation in my cervical spine. At the end of the episode, he told me to just go away and live life normally. Whatever happened might never happen again. Then my next neurologist said it was benign MS. He also said not to worry. It was my third neurologist who really told me what I had and started treatment. But that was years later.'

'Well, I'll say it again, I think you're doing really well.'

'Thanks. The thing that's funny is, sometimes I think getting MS was the best thing that happened to me. I had to stop work, so I was able to do all the many other things that I love doing, especially travelling. It's like I've lived two lives.'

Bob and Kerrie were good to chat with and we met up with them several times after that.

With another full day at sea ahead, we decided to check out a few more things on the ship and about the cruise.

I became aware that some optional excursions were available for when we got closer to the mainland. When I got hold of a list of the excursions in English, I saw that many of them were marked 'cancelled' or 'fully booked'.

'How can any of them be fully booked?' I asked. 'We've only just received this information.' The only answer I received was, 'You have to be quick, some of them fill up fast.'

I was relatively new to cruising. Our earlier trip to Antarctica had included everything in a package – all the outings, all the excursions were taken care of. I didn't realise that the details of the excursions on this trip were available well ahead of the cruise. I also didn't know that we could make bookings for them many months before we travelled. The travel agent hadn't told us this and I didn't think to ask.

Carolyn had given me a list of excursions from her trip, and I'd looked at those before we left. I'd thought I understood what she meant about being able to walk around towns on our own; I took that to mean we wouldn't need to be part of an excursion. The problem with that was we weren't going to most of the towns that Carolyn had gone to. I also wrongly assumed that they were optional extras that we probably wouldn't want or that many of them wouldn't be suitable for me. I didn't expect to be going on any excursions.

But when I looked at our excursion list, I saw that there were symbols against each one as a guide to the required level of fitness. Some had 'suitable for wheelchairs'.

There was one coming up the next day. It was a bus ride to Nordkapp. Carolyn had told me about that one. I remember her saying, 'That excursion is really worthwhile. You get to see the countryside, and there's even a stop to see a baby reindeer.' Sue would like that, I thought.

After discussing it with her, I wanted to book the Nordkapp bus trip straight away. But I had to wait until the next day for the booking desk to open.

The ship's team provided information daily. They posted it on the TV screens in the cabins and had it available in hard-copy printouts that were left in the bistro area. That day, I noticed an advertisement for an 'Additional surprise excursion offer, 14/9, Highlights of Trollfjord–Svolvær in a polar circle boat. Only bookable on board, not offered in any pre-trip material.'

It was an excursion for thirty-two participants, for one-and-a-half hours and went 'through narrow sounds in a very scenic area'. The cost was 640 kr and it was in three days' time on the Norwegian mainland.

Suddenly, the situation with excursions – the choices, the decisions and the bookings – hit me. How had I missed all of this? After dinner, we took the list of excursions and all the relevant paperwork back to the cabin with us. I wanted to study them that night, in case we wanted to book more than the Nordkapp trip the next day.

The ship spent the night and the next morning travelling south-east in the North Sea to reach the Norwegian mainland, 550 kilometres south-east of Spitsbergen.

I went to the booking desk after breakfast and was able to book the Nordkapp excursion. There were plenty of spaces left. We booked a few other excursions too. All that brief panic, though, was a good lesson, I thought. I'd have to remember to book the additional excursions before we left next time.

In the early afternoon of Cruise Day 5, we saw the cliffs of Nordkapp from the sea. Nordkapp, or North Cape, was the northernmost point of Norway's coastline. It was also the northernmost point of any mainland in the world.

There was a monument high up on a plateau. The cliffs were tall and steep going up to it. The ship sailed a little further north of the monument before turning around and heading back down south.

The next part of our expedition cruise had begun.

CHAPTER 4

NORWAY: CRUISE PART 2

It was the first time for our cruise to visit the Norwegian mainland. But we'd returned, this time at the very top, about two thousand kilometres north of Oslo. For the next eight days, we were going to travel south and visit places on the west coast of Norway. Our ship's schedule listed eleven stops. We began that part of our journey on 12 September, towards the end of Cruise Day 5.

Although it was late in afternoon, there was still a lot of light left in the day. Our first port of call was the town of Honningsvåg, just a little south of Nordkapp.

Our ship was to moor at a pier in the centre of town. As we approached, I could see that another Hurtigruten ship had arrived, the MS *King Harald*. I knew Honningsvåg was a port of call on the Norwegian coastal run. Carolyn's ship had been the MS *Midnatsol* when she was here months before. This was one place with a slightly familiar ring to it, and I could see that it must be a popular stop.

Honningsvåg is a small town of around 2,500 people, with brightly painted buildings of yellow, white, Scandinavian red and grey. The town is set at the base of hills and mountains, right on the water. The buildings are mostly three storeys high and huddled together, but with some grass and trees between them. Grass covers parts of the hills and mountains behind the town too, while other sections are just bare rock.

The green colour surprised me. For days, we'd been looking

at white or black on any land we'd passed. Later, I learned about the warm Gulf Stream that flows past Honningsvåg. It creates a warmer subarctic climate where grasses can grow, quite different to where we'd come from.

After our ship arrived, there were announcements saying that buses were ready for us. There were two bus excursions, one to Nordkapp and the other to 'Taste the King Crab'.

We disembarked, going down the ramp from Deck Level 3. Sue rolled the scooter down and I walked with my stick, using the handrail for additional support. I got on the scooter at the base of the ramp and we went over to the buses parked nearby. Attendants directed us to the right bus and the scooter went into the lower luggage compartment. I could step up into the bus using its handrail and my stick. There were two more steps up after the landing, and then I made my way to a spare seat. There were two or three buses going to Nordkapp that day. We had about two hundred people on board our ship and most of them went on this excursion.

On the way to Nordkapp, the buses stopped at a 'Sami cultural experience' spot. There was a reindeer and people dressed in traditional Sami clothing in a small fenced-in area. There was a tent (it looked like a wigwam), the frame of an old fishing boat, an old saw and some other objects from past times. An older man, in Sami dress and a hat, stood next to the reindeer for photos. Some women, also traditionally dressed, were just outside a wooden shelter, selling what looked like souvenirs inside.

The buses parked outside the small fenced-in area. 'It looks like it's going to rain,' said Sue after getting up and looking around. 'Do you really want to go out there?'

The weather had suddenly changed. 'No, I'll stay here.' I had a window seat and could see everything that was going on outside. It started to rain, and it looked cold and bleak outside.

The whole area was wild and barren. There'd been very few houses along the way and there were none here either. Then I noticed a small house opposite the fenced area on the other side of the road. I wondered if the family lived there or perhaps used it as a place to stay warm, while waiting for tourists to arrive. I thought that perhaps when they knew some tourists were coming, they could quickly put on their traditional clothes and run across the road. Perhaps it was just a large comfy changing room.

Everyone else got off the bus and I saw people taking photos. I took one or two photos too, but I thought it was all a bit sad, a bit of a set-up, too touristy. The big reindeer was the first animal we'd seen since the polar bears. I didn't see any baby reindeer, but the large, older reindeer had wonderful big antlers. It was eating something and was tied to an old sled beside the tent. The baby must have grown up and gone somewhere else in the three months since Carolyn had seen it.

I was pleased that I'd already read something about the culture of the Sami in the Oslo museums, and that I'd learned about the Lapps and Lapland when I was a child. I found out later that the Sami people preferred the name 'Sami' to 'Lapp'. Their people first arrived in northern Scandinavia eleven thousand years ago. They were Norway's indigenous people.

I thought the Samis must have a lot in common with Native Americans, who also used wigwam tents. I saw those tents in American western movies. 'Conquering the wild west,' they said. I reflected on how poorly the movies told that story. *Lavvo* was the Sami word for a tent. What a different way of living it must have been in those tents, and there I was, sitting in a warm bus looking out at one.

With everyone back on the bus, we continued on to Nordkapp. The whole journey from the ship only took about forty minutes. At our destination, we stopped at a large building set on a plateau with a metal monument on the other side, facing the ocean near a cliff face. There was a sign out the front that said 'Nordkapp N71°10'21'. The rain had stopped.

The large building spread out over several levels. Inside, there were lifts and access everywhere was easy. There was a large cinema, a restaurant, a post office and shops selling clothes and souvenirs.

They had laid everything out well, geared apparently for the thousands of tourists who came each year. Tickets to the cinema were included in our excursion. We filed in and watched a 'short educational panoramic film across five screens in a 120° theatre'. The film was all about that area of Norway. It was a good film, I thought, and I learned a lot.

After the film, I was keen to get outside and go over to the edge of the cliff. I wanted to capture the view before the light faded. It was windy and a bit wild. The surface of the ground was composed of thickly laid gravel and small stones. It wasn't suitable for my scooter. The wheels sank down and stopped moving. I parked the scooter near the glass exit doors and walked out with my stick, holding on to Sue's arm very firmly. I sank into the ground too, making me even slower.

There was a fence along the top of the cliff face and the views from there were spectacular. It was so far north and the sun was trying to get down below the horizon in the west. The clouds were amazing too, appearing in all sorts of formations. I took lots of photos and stood watching for a while. I was in awe of the wild landscape.

The monument near the edge of the cliff was made of sculptured metal and overlooked the Barents Sea. It was the same monument I'd seen earlier that day from the ship. It was a large, round, metal representation of a globe, held up by legs splayed on to an elevated concrete slab, with steps up. I looked at it from a distance.

Back inside the building, and on the scooter again, I felt lovely and warm. We took the lift to a lower level via a stop at the toilets. The disabled toilet was excellent. Below the building was a passageway through the rock leading out to the ocean. The passageway led to some odd areas – a Thai museum and St Johannes Chapel. I didn't spend much time looking at them but moved quickly past to get to the end where I thought there might be another view. There was.

A small viewing area jutted out at the end of the passageway. From there, I imagined I could see across to the top of the world –

the watery North Pole. I looked down at the ocean waves crashing three hundred metres below. Once again, the clouds in the unusual sky were stunning and there were so many of them. They made the sky look darker, as though it were later in the day than it really was. The whole place seemed special.

After soaking in the views for a bit longer, it was time to leave. My scooter was perfect inside the building and also out on the driveway. We went back to the buses with everyone else.

As we were driving back to the ship, I saw two white reindeer with antlers, munching plants in the hills. The photos I took all turned out to be blurry, but it didn't matter; I enjoyed seeing the reindeer in the wild.

Back in our cabin on the ship, I noted once again the ship's location on the TV map. We really were on the northernmost tip of the mainland near Nordkapp. (Photo 3.4.1)

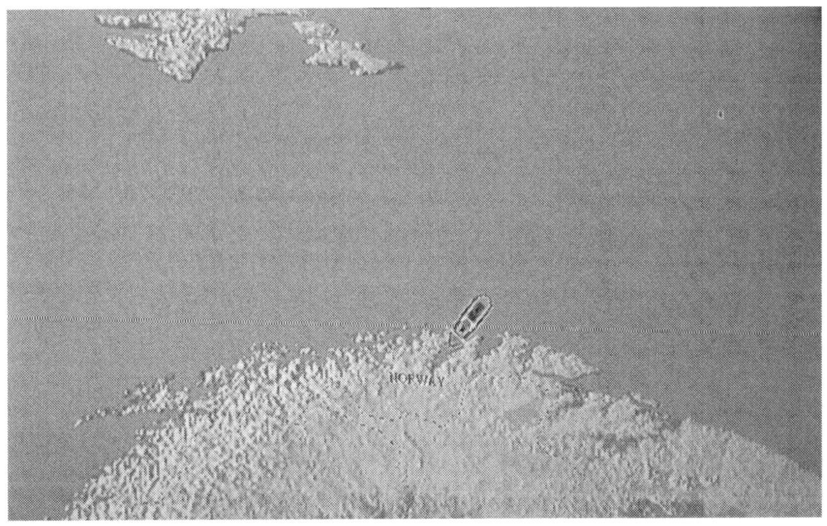

Photo 3.4.1 Map of ship at Honningsvåg near Nordkapp

Our first mainland excursion had worked out well. The next wheelchair-suitable excursion was at Tromsø the next day. It was a cable-car trip.

We arrived at Tromsø early in the morning of Cruise Day 6.

The sun had risen but the morning mist was still hanging in the air. I was out on the observation terrace as we approached a long bridge arching over our path. It was a beautiful sight. To my right, I could see three large ski-jump structures, sitting side by side near the top of a small hill. They were behind some high-rise buildings of five or six storeys, all waiting for snow. After we went under the bridge, I could see the Arctic Cathedral on my left, with the cable car and its cables going up the mountain behind it.

Tromsø is the only city in northern Norway. It sits on an island linked by two large arching bridges to the mainland. Tromsø has a population of about 65,000 people and is almost four hundred kilometres north of the Arctic Circle. The warm Gulf Stream just about reaches this point too and helps keep the temperatures higher than you might expect at this latitude.

After the ship moored near the city centre, we went out to the bus. We started the excursion with a guided tour of the city of Tromsø.

Different activities happened in the Tromsø region throughout the year, from a midnight sun marathon to summer hiking and winter dog sledding. Our guide told us about the history of Tromsø, how it used to be the place where polar discovery expeditions started. Tromsø was also the home of the Northern Lights. The guide said there was a chance that, over the next two nights, we might be able to see them. 'That is,' he said, 'if there are no clouds in the night sky.' It was an exciting possibility. I must keep a watch out tonight for sure, I thought.

The bus stopped at the bottom of a mountain. Sue and I got off and, with the driver's help, Sue unloaded the scooter from the lower compartment. There was a queue of people going up a flight of stairs, many in the same blue jackets as us, from a bus that had arrived a bit earlier. Sue went ahead and checked the route. She came back and said, 'There are even more stairs inside. I've asked the tour guide and he said he doesn't know any other way to get on to the cable car. He's offered to lift the scooter up there.'

'So much for selecting a "suitable for wheelchairs" excursion,' I said. How would we handle this one? I was going to give it a go, as my mother would say.

There was quite a lot of waiting around. The cable car could hold about ten people and there seemed to be only one operating. Perhaps there were two, but there were easily fifty people waiting. It seemed to take at least thirty to forty minutes to get in. Our guide carried the scooter up to the entry level.

I walked up the steps slowly, one by one. Sue found a chair for me to sit on at the halfway point. I chatted with Bruce and Helen from the ship. They told me a bit more about where they lived in Colorado and what they did there.

Once I reached the top of the two sets of stairs, I thought I'd be able to get on my scooter and ride into the cable car. But there wasn't enough room. I could see that if I went in on my scooter, there'd only be enough room for a couple of other people. So, instead, I walked into it, holding Sue's arm. Our guide followed us, with the scooter collapsed and upright at 90° to its usual position.

There was a small bench seat at either end of the cable car. People kindly moved aside and let me sit on one. The cable car went above trees displaying autumn colours, and the view was lovely. When we reached the top and got out, there was another very long, narrow staircase going up to the viewing area. Wow, this is incredible! I thought. More stairs! I let the others go first and then climbed the stairs slowly.

I don't recall seeing a handrail; there was just the wall and my stick. It was very slow-going and a big effort for me. I might even have thought about the 'not very big' Little Blue Engine pulling the little train that had broken down in the wonderful children's book, *The Little Engine That Could*. I will never forget some of the stories that Mum used to read to me when I was a child. The Little Blue Engine trying to get up the hill said, 'I think I can. I think I can…' then, 'I thought I could. I thought I could…' I am sure that mum would have added, 'Yes you can, you know you can, yes you can. You can do it.'

While I climbed the stairs, the guide carried my scooter up to the next level again. Both Sue and I were becoming quite cranky by this stage. We mentioned the wheelchair-suitable note to the guide. He said he didn't know anything about that.

I felt very tired by the time I got to the top. Sue put my scooter into working order and I scooted out to look at the view and have a rest. I was soon happily taking photos. I could see the two arching bridges and the Arctic Cathedral. The cathedral had multiple inverted white Vs that formed the roof. It really stood out.

From that high up, the views of the waterways were stunning, and the snow-capped mountains surrounding them made for a perfect picture. I could also see our ship moored in the harbour. I zoomed to 550 millimetres to take a photo including the ship. There was so much around me to look at. The two arched bridges linking the sections of land in the middle were especially striking.

I took note of one very interesting building in the city below. From up there, high on the mountain, it looked like six white books stacked against each other, with their spines clinging on to the land and their pages opening away from the water. I learned later that this was part of a building called the Polaria – Tromsø's museum of the Arctic.

Our guide soon called us to return to the bus. We went down the same way that we came up, except I got to miss the short set of stairs at the bottom; the bus driver met us and showed us another way out. It was out the other side of the entrance and around the building down a ramp. At least that small section was a wheelchair-friendly discovery. Gee whiz, wouldn't it have made things a bit easier if that was pointed out to me in the beginning, I thought. Or maybe I should have asked the bus driver. Anyway, I made it, I did it, and the view was worth it.

On the way back to the ship, the bus stopped to let us visit the Arctic Cathedral. We got off and I went inside easily on the ramps at the entrance. I was still recovering from walking up the stairs so I stayed on my scooter.

When I was leaving and going down the ramp on my scooter, I noticed a man leaning on the rail using a camera with a label on it that read '16x Zoom'. He seemed like a nice, friendly fellow. I said, 'Mine is 26x zoom,' and pointed to the numbers on my camera.

He laughed and said, 'That's really good.' Nothing else. We smiled at each other and moved on.

I took a few more photos outside while sitting on my scooter. I didn't feel like standing up. There was some nice warm bright sunshine and the waterways with the mountains behind them looked very scenic. I could also see our ship moored again. I took another photo of it – I couldn't help myself! It was moored near the centre of Tromsø, with shops and buildings surrounding it. Green fir trees were scattered among houses on a small hill and snow-topped mountains rose in the distance. It was very beautiful.

After the Arctic Cathedral, the bus took us back to the ship. There was still plenty of time left in the day. We had lunch in the ship's restaurant.

After lunch, we got off the ship again and went for a walk through Tromsø. It was a lovely small city and very pretty. There were flowers in baskets hanging in the streets and in front of shops. The buildings were wooden, three storeys, with shop windows at street level. The main street had become a pedestrian mall. It was easy to walk and scooter.

I wondered where the cars were. There were a few cars in the streets behind the mall, but not many. I noticed an arched entrance into the side of a hill in one of the back streets. It looked dark inside. Then I read the sign above the arch: 'Tromsø *parkering*'. A car with its headlights on came out. That's where they were. It was so unlike our high-rise car parks in Australia.

In the streets surrounding the mall, we went past two old churches. The main one was Tromsø Domkirke and the sign on it indicated that it was built in 1861. It was the Church of Norway's Tromsø cathedral and one of Norway's largest wooden churches. There were many other early nineteenth-century timber buildings too. The other church in the city was a smaller Catholic one. The Catholic religion had never had a large following in Norway.

I'd read about an interesting museum of art in Tromsø. The

street map in my *Lonely Planet Norway* showed me the way to this place, the Nordnorsk Kunstmuseum. There was a ramp up to the entry door.

The museum was in an old four-storey stone and brick building containing many different galleries. There were galleries for sculpture, photography and paintings. We wandered into all of them but we spent most of our time with the paintings.

Most of the work in the museum was by artists from northern Norway. However, there was one painting by a Norwegian from further south – Edvard Munch. His painting *The Scream* is famous; it's in the Munch Museum in Oslo. We didn't get to visit that museum while we were there, and I've only seen pictures of *The Scream*. It's unforgettable. The painting in the museum in Tromsø was also striking but quite different. It was much simpler, of a woman dressed in a blouse and skirt, standing with her hands together in front of her, expressionless.

Back near our ship at the end of our day in Tromsø, I noticed the MS *Midnatsol*, the Hurtigruten ship that Carolyn had been on in June. It was moored just behind us.

There was still a little bit more of Stortorget Harbour to see, so we wandered further along. There were a lot of fishing boats moored there, making fantastic reflections in the water. The arched bridge was often behind them and the sky was so blue. Tufts of fluffy white clouds were perfectly reflected in the water. I really enjoyed looking at these scenes and enjoyed myself even more by taking lots of photos as we went along.

The headquarters of the Hurtigruten line are in Tromsø, and most of the ships calling there belonged to them. But it was new for the MS *Fram* to be there. It usually spent its time in more remote places.

In our daily information sheets, there was a note saying that some of the land-based Hurtigruten staff from Tromsø would be coming onboard throughout the day to see the ship. They seemed very friendly, and they were happy and excited to be touring the MS *Fram*.

Before our ship left Tromsø, we went up to the observation lounge on Deck 7. We found some nice comfy chairs and decided to have a glass of white wine before dinner. We watched the MS *Midnatsol* leave. It went under the bridge and out between some islands to continue its route. It was still light as we watched it disappear.

There was one more announcement at Tromsø. The man with the broken bones who'd been rescued by helicopter was returning to the ship. We were told he'd broken his wrist in several places and had been in hospital, but was now fit enough to continue with us. We all clapped our hands to welcome him back.

We left not long after and went into the waters between some islands, still close to the mainland coast, heading south. We looked out of the windows into the sky many times that night, hoping to see coloured lights. But there were too many clouds. So I didn't see the Northern Lights. I thought I'd just have to come back another time.

We were headed to the Lofoten Islands. They were supposed to be absolutely beautiful. They formed an archipelago that stretched out like the end of a long drooping finger from the Norwegian mainland. I remembered Carolyn telling me that the Norwegian government was committed to preserving the culture and lifestyle of the small villages on the islands by keeping them all linked to the mainland. 'There are bridges between them all,' explained Carolyn. 'It makes transport easy so the little places can survive.'

While we were having breakfast the next day, Cruise Day 7, I realised that we were almost there. We went through the top end of the archipelago, along a very scenic passage between Vesterålen and Lofoten. It was gentle sailing, and we passed close by mountains and hills on the way through. Lone fishermen's cottages appeared here and there, with short piers and small boats nearby. I was soon up and out on deck to soak it all in.

We came to an open area with a narrow pass ahead. The pass led into a fjord where waterfalls flowed over cliffs, rocks and green grasses into still blue waters. The ship moored nearby.

I sat on the deck with Thilli and Anni. The warmth of the sun was coming down nicely and we were feeling relaxed, looking out at the beautiful landscape around us. There wasn't much conversation until Thilli asked me a question. 'If you do not mind, what field of work were you in?'

I thought about my response for a short time and then answered. 'I was a doctor.'

There was a sharp intake of breath from both of them. 'What kind?'

'A medical doctor. I mostly worked in management and administration. I was a GP first and then went back to university to get qualifications in management. I worked in hospitals and health services.'

'And Sue, is she a nurse?'

'No, she's not.'

'Oh, it's just that she looks after you as if she has some knowledge and knows what to do.'

An announcement interrupted our conversation; it was about the 'additional surprise excursion' to Trollfjord and Svolvær that they'd told us about when we were at Bear Island a few days ago. We were now at the mouth of Trollfjord. Some people started getting off the ship and into the polar circle boats. To my mind, those boats were really just big dinghies, but they were calling it a 'boat cruise'.

We watched people stepping off a platform at the bottom of the set of steps going down the side of the ship and into the boats. The ship's crew had put the steps out not long before and lowered the boats into the water ready for the excursion. We waved to Glenda; she was sitting in a boat. Sue said, 'Gee, you have to give it to her. Glenda is into everything, isn't she? I think she's fantastic.'

'Yes, she sure is.'

The boats went forward and the ship followed behind for a while. We watched them out the front of us and then saw them at our side as we overtook them. They were very close to the rocks and waterfalls in that narrow passageway. We were soon all in the passageway that led south-west, away from the mouth of Trollfjord, past some of the Lofoten Islands, and on to the sea on the other side. It was very scenic indeed.

The waters on the other side of the archipelago were calm and warm. They were protected from the cold ocean currents by the islands. Codfish came from the Barents Sea in winter to spawn there. We were entering an area of great cod fisheries. We went past fishing cottages, farmhouses, sheltered bays and sheep in pastures. Spectacular rural scenery, I thought.

As we were nearing our next destination, I saw wooden drying racks near the edge of the water. When we were closer, I could see that the racks were empty. The cod had finished drying long ago.

I learned that most of the commercial fishing in the area was of stockfish, especially cod, with tonnes of them decapitated, paired by size and tied together. The fishermen would leave them dangling in pairs to dry over the wooden A-frames.

There was a statue at the entrance to the harbour of a woman holding her hand high in the air and waving. She was farewelling and greeting the men who went out to sea to fish.

Our ship moored at a pier in the port town of Svolvær. This was our third stop and it was Cruise Day 7, 14 September. There were brightly coloured apartment buildings that looked like holiday accommodation by the harbour's waters. They would have had views of the snow-dusted mountains at the other end of the town. There were many empty A-frame drying racks about as well. At the end of March each year, there was a Cod Fishing Championship in Svolvær. Perhaps these apartments were where visitors stayed.

There was a bus waiting at the pier. It was the shuttle bus service organised for our ship. It was running from Svolvær to Henningsvær and back.

As the bus went out into the countryside along the coast and over a few bridges, the weather changed. It became very windy and rainy. It took about forty-five minutes to get to Henningsvær. The bus parked on the edge of the little village in a large asphalt parking area. I got off the bus and on to my scooter, which had, as always, been loaded into the lower luggage area of the bus. The driver helped Sue.

I scootered past several dried cod hanging from the roof of a shed as we went into the centre of the village. They'd had their heads cut off and were tied together in pairs, just as I'd read. They were hanging in front of the timber wall of the shed, and the wood was painted in that typical Scandinavian red. I took a photo of a few pairs. I thought they'd make a good symbol of the whole area, to remember it by. (Photo 3.4.2)

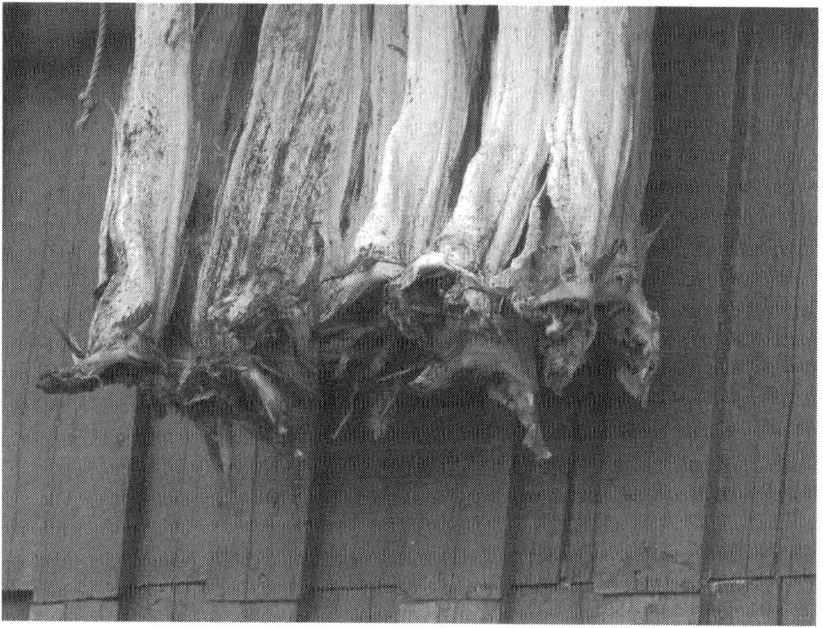

Photo 3.4.2 Hanging codfish at Henningsvær

Everything in the village, except the souvenir shop, was closed. We went out on to a wharf to get a bit of the sun that was coming through the clouds. I could see that all the little wooden houses were arranged in a semi-circle around a small harbour.

While I was on the wharf, looking about and thinking, Thilli came up to me and said, 'We have a problem.'

'What is it?' I replied quickly.

'We have no money. We left the ship and we both forgot to bring cash. We want to buy some things at the souvenir shop and it is closing soon. Could you lend us a small amount, please?'

'Oh, that's no problem,' I said and called out to Sue. She usually carried the cash because she was upright most of the time and she could put her hands into her pockets to get money out more easily than I could.

Sue came over and I explained. Sue took out the cash she had (only €20) and gave it to Thilli.

'Oh, thank you, we will give you back the money when we are on the ship again.'

'Sure, no worries.'

Thilli and Anni went into the souvenir shop. Sue and I continued to walk around the deserted little town in the strong wind. The sun was gone and after about another five minutes we decided we'd rush back and get the same bus to the ship. If we didn't go back on the same bus, we'd have to wait over an hour for it to come back again. There was also nowhere sheltered to wait if we didn't make it.

We went as fast as we could and just made it to the bus, where it was warm inside, and went back to the ship. When I saw postcards of Henningsvær later, it looked such a lovely place with the sun out, shops and restaurants open and people about. It showed a nice harbour with mountains in the background. It didn't look like that when we saw it. Weather can change everything, I thought.

I was also glad that we went back to the ship when we did. We were able to board using the ramp again, but, after that time, there was boarding only by tender boat. The tender boats weren't difficult, but it was just easier to walk up the ramp on to the ship using the rail. They had to use tender boats because the Hurtigruten MS *Trollfjord* was arriving at Svolvær on its coastal run and our ship had to vacate its spot.

Whenever two Hurtigruten ships passed each other they gave a loud hoot of their horns to say hello. We'd experienced that a few times already and it happened once again when MS *Trollfjord* arrived.

After our buffet dinner that night, we went back to our cabin and the ship continued to sail south.

The next day, we were going to be in Helgeland on our eighth day of cruising. The ship crossed the Arctic Circle at 66°33'N early in the morning, well south of the main Lofoten islands.

I was trying to locate where we were on my maps. The Lofoten chain of islands was a landmark and a prominent feature on any map of Norway. The drooping finger projected out west and then south off the coast. All I had to do was locate them, look east back to the mainland and then go south of that. But I couldn't see where we were going next marked on any of my maps.

I knew it would be difficult to remember exactly where I'd taken photos. But I made sure I included a sign as often as I could in the sequence to help. The photos were numbered but the signs really helped.

There were so many places. I didn't appreciate how many there'd be before we left. I had a tour schedule, the ship's information sheets and my own travel table. With all the different numbers of days, stops and landings, I realised that I had mixed up some of the numbers on my original table. I had to make up another table much later to help me remember where I really was (Appendix 3)!

After a while, I was enjoying the trip so much that I just let everything flow. The numbers didn't matter that much. My maps weren't good enough to pick up exactly where we were going anyway, and with the myriad of islands, rocks and fjords, I found it easy to be quite lost at times.

On the way to breakfast the next morning, there was an announcement to look out from the portside (the left) to see the Seven Sisters, a formation of several mountains close together. I looked, but I couldn't see any mountains. The Seven Sisters were a landmark in this area, in the waters of Alstahaug. But I missed the Sisters.

Alstahaug is a municipality of more than nine hundred islands grouped together. It's part of the Helgeland collection of thousands of islands in the shallow waters off the coast. The whole of Helgeland had pointed mountains and *strandflaten* – shallow lowland areas, sometimes just above sea level and sometimes just below. That was a new word to me and I liked it.

We were going to one of the islands. To get on to it, we had to go from the ship by polar circle boat. Alstahaug would be our fourth stop.

I didn't leave the ship to explore Alstahaug. When I asked about the paths on the island, I found out there weren't really any. The walk would be on dirt paths and across grass and hills – not suitable for my yellow Luggie scooter. If I'd had my grey Parmaker scooter, it certainly would have been suitable. But that's too heavy to take on overseas trips and it was at home. My yellow Luggie scooter really was the best for travelling and most of the time it had been perfect.

I watched all the activities happening outside. The island in front of me looked like a very small place with only a few buildings on it. I saw Thilli and Anni going over in their boat and I also saw Sue in hers. I took photos of them all. I thought Thilli and Anni would like copies of the photos of themselves so I took one for them. Through my superzoom lens, I followed Sue's boat to a metal floating pier with a ramp up and over to the island. Zooming in with the camera lens made for a good set of binoculars sometimes.

Alstahaug was in the 'kingdom of Petter Dass'. He was a famous Norwegian church minister, poet and writer who lived here in the late 1600s and early 1700s. There was a church and a museum on the island. The museum looked very modern. The building rose out of the land to project over the water. On the side facing the water, it was all glass, while the other sides were metal. It was right on the water's edge and architecturally striking. It must have been built recently, I thought.

All the boats had finished transferring people to the island, and it was so peaceful and quiet on the ship as it gently sat in those waters. It seemed very fitting to be near a church, a place of contemplation. I could just see the church spire from the ship. Apparently, it dated back to the year 1200.

When Sue came back she said, 'I couldn't get into the museum. They were only allowing people on the booked excursion to go in. Apparently, there was a seminar going on and they didn't want too many visitors. Shame. It seemed as if it might have been interesting.'

Other than the museum, Sue told me that the place was a bit like a farm, with just a few buildings. 'You wouldn't have been able to get around. It was rough walking and there was one little hill, all grass and dirt, just as they said. It was only a very small place. But there were horses there, baby horses. I videoed them.' Sue loves animals, especially baby ones.

Petter Dass was an important cultural figure in Norway. He was a Lutheran pastor and his writings were religious and connected to the land of Northern Norway. He wrote baroque hymns and 'topographical poetry'. I'd never heard of the latter. I thought I must look that up one day. There was no Wi-Fi on the ship so I couldn't look it up then. But I didn't feel like trying to look up anything anyway. It sounded like something connected to the landscape, and I preferred to just look out from the ship and think about the place.

The only sources of information on the cruise were books and conversation. It was internet- and Google-free. It wasn't too bad at all, I thought, using those old-fashioned ways. And there was plenty of time for a good old think as well. In fact, I couldn't remember having Googled anything since I left home.

Everyone was back on board by about noon, and we left Alstahaug just as lunch was about to be served. When we went into the dining room Sue said, 'Why don't we sit with those two Japanese women? There's no one else at their table over there near the window. I've noticed them a few times. They seem to keep to themselves a lot.'

'Sure, what a good idea,' I said.

We said hello to the two Japanese women and checked that the free seats weren't for someone else. After a little while we were all chatting. One woman was much older than the other. We learned that their husbands had been very good friends and professional colleagues. They'd both died. The older woman's husband had died most recently and she was so upset that she was doing a lot of travelling to help her cope with her grief.

The younger woman spoke some English and the older one spoke none at all. The younger one translated our questions and answers back and forth. She explained what had happened to their husbands and that the two of them had teamed up to travel together.

Not long after I'd told them that I was a doctor, in the course of the conversation, the older woman asked me about influenza vaccinations. The younger woman told me that her friend had been doing some research and had gone to Tasmania to give a lecture. Her husband had been a well-known medical man in Japan.

'What do you think of the flu vaccine?' the older woman asked me through her friend.

'I think it's very good. I have a flu shot every year,' I answered enthusiastically.

'No, it is bad. Not good.'

'Oh, umm…,' I said, and stopped talking about that. I wasn't sure if we were talking about the same thing and I didn't think we'd be able to communicate about it in any meaningful way. So I changed the subject. We'd finished lunch by then, anyway. Otherwise, we enjoyed having lunch with the two of them, chatting as best we could in spite of the language barrier.

Sue asked me later what was said in the conversation because she'd missed it. She'd only picked up that the older woman didn't seem very happy with what I'd said. 'You're as blunt as a tack sometimes but what you said doesn't seem too bad.'

'Well, she asked me and I told her. It's a fact, isn't it?'

'Maybe she didn't understand. Or maybe she just has her own opinion.'

'Oh well. I hope I didn't upset her for whatever reason. They seemed to be very nice people.'

After lunch, we arrived at Vega, our fifth stop, also on Cruise Day 8. Vega was the largest island in the Vega Archipelago. It's home to eider ducks, whose feathers are used for making eiderdown. There was an excursion to go and see them. Sue and I didn't go, but Thilli and Anni did.

The ship moored out in the bay, and Sue and I decided that we'd go to the shore by polar circle boat for a walk around the area. I was thrilled that my scooter fitted into the boat without any problems. Of all the times I'd been off the ship so far, this was the first stop where I'd got the scooter on to land without using the ramp. It all happened so quickly and easily. After it was collapsed down, the crew helped Sue load it on to the boat. We were at the shore in no time at all and a crew member unloaded the scooter for us at the other end.

There was a jetty on the landing that had a good surface on which to scooter. Then there were roads and a few paths. But there wasn't really much to see. It was good to be off the ship, though, and walking in the countryside.

Thinking of Mum's postcard, I took some photos of grass growing on rooftops as well as some of the reflections of several old fishing sheds in the water. This was my attempt to create an artistic picture to put somewhere at home.

Thilli and Anni sought us out that night to give us a collection of gifts along with the €20 they'd borrowed. There was a serviette with a map on it of where their excursion had gone that day. Loving maps, I was happily surprised when I was given one on a serviette! I'd never seen that before. How nice, I thought, quite different.

There was also a heart-shaped chocolate and pictures from their excursion. They explained what they'd learned about the eider ducks. Thilli told us that those families whose business it had been for many generations to look after these special ducks, loved and cared for them. The duck families had their own special houses. Thilli and Anni showed us brochures with photos of the duck houses.

In a brochure about the Vega Archipelago, I read that it was one of the seven Norwegian UNESCO World Heritage Sites. I'd had no idea. The Vega Archipelago was added to the World Heritage List in 2004. The committee thought that 'the Vega Archipelago reflects the way generations of fishermen/farmers have, over the past 1,500 years, maintained a sustainable living in an inhospitable seascape near the Arctic Circle, based on the now unique practice of eider down harvesting, and it also celebrates the contribution made by women to the eider down process.'

I wondered about all the rocks and small islands that we were cruising past. The brochure helped me understand. It said that parts of the Norwegian west coast are fringed by *strandflaten*. There was that word again. The brochure said, 'A strandflat coast typically consists of numerous low islands and scattered coastal peaks' and 'the World Heritage Area contains more than 6,500 islands, islets and skerries.' I'd heard of skerries – they were rocks in the sea. There certainly seemed to be a lot of rocks and rocky islands everywhere. It's a wonder the ship doesn't run into one was the thought that flashed through my mind.

The brochure listed seven Norwegian World Heritage Sites. The sites were numbered one to seven, going from north to south, with Vega being number three. Number five was the West Norwegian Fjords. That was where our Nutshell trip was going to be. There was no mention of any particular fjord, such as Nærøyfjord. But I didn't let that worry me.

I enjoyed reading all the information that Thilli and Anni gave us. They seemed very appreciative of our small loan. We met up with them again from time to time and went out on a few walks together. They belonged to some walking groups back home in Germany. They loved walking, and Sue and I loved walking too.

After Vega, we continued south. We left the districts of North Norway and entered Central Norway, sailing into the Trøndelag region. Our next stop was in the Ørland municipality, at its administrative capital Brekstad. It was Friday, 16 September, our sixth stop, on Cruise Day 9. Our destination was near the large city of Trondheim, but we weren't going there.

Once again, we were in a fjord within a fjord. Brekstad, a small city of about two thousand people, was located on Trondheimsfjord at the entrance to the Stjørnfjord.

'There is an old church that would be interesting to see at Brekstad,' said Thilli. 'Do you want to walk there with us? We could all go together.'

'Yes, that sounds good,' I replied.

'What time should we meet? Where will we meet?'

We agreed on a time and met on the pier on land. The ship had moored offshore again and we used the polar circle boats to get to the pier.

The small pier was directly in front of a hotel on the waterfront of Brekstad. Some of the passengers on our ship were going to the 'gourmet food of the region tasting' at the hotel as a luncheon excursion. We moved through the area where the event was being set up to get out into the town streets behind it. We went out past the city library. The library was part of the set of buildings where the hotel was located. It all seemed quite recently built.

Out on the main street, the four of us turned right – I think that was north, or it could have been south! – up past the shops. I didn't have a map and was following the other three. A vegetable vendor had set up a table under an umbrella up ahead. Sue stopped to look. Thilli and Anni joined her. I was happy taking photos of all that was about me, including of them talking vegetables with the local woman.

Thilli had a town map and directed us to turn left when we reached the end of the street. '*Links*,' she said. We were starting to learn German.

The church was up the road and over an open grassy area. A cemetery surrounded the old white building and a metal flag on top of the steeple was marked '1893'. The gravestones were interesting, some of them were hundreds of years old. The graves were in a park-like setting with tall trees scattered around. They were different to graves back home, and it wasn't just the language. There seemed to be a slightly different attitude to death and burial here. The atmosphere was calm, welcoming and reassuring. It was a pleasant place. There were some seats, a table and a flower garden. I felt I could happily and easily just sit there and think for a while.

I didn't know a cemetery could be like that.

Thilli had gone ahead. She came back and said disappointedly, 'The church is closed and the door is locked. We can't go in.'

We left the church and found our way back to the ship by going around the other side of the tiny city. There was only one main street, a few hundred metres long, with the shops leading to the church, and only a few back roads around houses and along fields on the other side of the town.

On the way, I could smell something strong in the air. I looked about and saw a large wooden shed with a ramp going up into the rear. All the doors and windows were closed and there was no one about. Then a woman walked past. I stopped her and asked, 'Can you please tell me what that shed is used for?'

'It is for the animals, it is nearly winter now,' she said.

Her English was good and we talked to her a little about where we were from and what we were doing there. I'd forgotten that farm animals lived in sheds during the winter in cold countries. That was the cause of the smell, then!

We continued down the road back to the harbour. Our ship lay anchored in the distance. Directly in front of us was a big wharf where ferries came and went carrying people and cars. There was a large bitumen area for cars and other vehicles to park, queue or drive through. I'd missed all of that before when we were walking up into the town.

I stopped to photograph one large ferry coming in. It had 'Trondheim' written on the side. I got a bit carried away taking photos and enjoying the scenes of water, islands and rocks. Thilli and Anni said they were going back to the ship and that they'd meet us at the pier to catch the boat back together. 'Sure, see you there, then,' I said.

Not long after that, I suddenly felt the urge to go to the toilet. I said to Sue, 'I need to go to the toilet. Do you remember seeing one in those buildings as we went through?'

'I'm not sure. Let's go and have a look this way,' said Sue. She walked towards a different entrance off the harbour into the buildings. We saw an ordinary toilet sign well into the building and then a disabled toilet sign not far away.

I went into the disabled toilet. By then, I was starting to think too much about it and I could feel my urge incontinence starting to kick in.

***

Whenever that happens, I try to distract my mind by doing mental arithmetic or by focusing on an object or a marking to try to stop my mind thinking about passing urine. The urge always gets worse the closer I get to the toilet bowl. I look around at the tiles, thinking to myself, count the tiles, count the tiles… 1, 2, 3, 4… Count the tiles. Subtract from 100 in 7s – 93, 86… Focus on that mark… Think of the mark… Think of the mark.

Urge incontinence is a funny thing about MS. As soon as I start to think about going to the toilet, I start going. Or, when I get into a familiar place where I know there's a toilet and where I have some mental association with going to the toilet, I might start going.

During my last year of working, whenever I'd driven my car home at the end of the day and parked it in the garage, my brain switched on to a pathway that said, Home. Toilet nearby. And I'd start to go. It happened just about every time. I'd have to force myself to think about something else – counting, maths puzzles – anything a little difficult. I tried to break the association and put my thoughts on a different mental pathway. After all, I thought, it was all in my head, or, rather, my brain and my nerve pathways. I was trying to re-educate and re-direct the process. Most times it worked but sometimes it didn't.

***

That time in Brekstad was one of the occasions when my distraction attempts failed.

I spent much longer in the toilet than usual. After some time, I went out to join Sue, who had been to the other toilet and was waiting patiently outside. I explained what had happened even though she probably knew already.

We headed back further inside the building to find another route to the pier and go back to the ship. We found a way that linked up with the way we'd come out earlier and followed it back. In the hotel lobby, they were tasting aquavit – 'Only Norwegian aquavit', they advertised. That was interesting, I thought. I hadn't heard of Norwegian aquavit, only Swedish.

When we finally reached the boats, Thilli and Anni weren't there. We assumed that they must have gone back to the ship without us. We hadn't been able to tell them that we'd been delayed. It would've been a bit difficult to explain anyway.

It was harder getting out to the pier than I remembered. There was a lot of loose gravel around, and it seemed a lot looser than earlier. Or maybe I was tired. I found a firm trail and once I arrived at the pier, I rode my scooter along the wooden boards and stopped where the boat was loading.

We collapsed the scooter down and a member of the crew helped Sue load it into the boat. There were steps and a handrail that folded out to help me get on. We were soon seated and whizzed back safely to the ship.

When we caught up with Thilli and Anni much later, they didn't say anything and neither did we.

Later that day, there was a notice sent out announcing that tomorrow there would be another 'additional excursion offer, only available on board and not available in any pre-trip material'. I hadn't seen any pre-trip material anyway, and the next day we were going to the famous Geirangerfjord. That was the same place as on Mum's postcard. She'd written it on 9 September 1984, just a few days before exactly twenty-seven years ago.

The additional excursion was a 'unique hike' to a famous farm, the notice said, in the mountainside of Geirangerfjord. It was going to be a very steep, mountainous walk for experienced hikers, taking three to three-and-a-half hours in the afternoon. I remembered the steep mountains on the postcard. I, of course, couldn't take up that offer, and Sue, with her bad knee, wasn't interested. But I was very keen to see it all happening.

There were a lot of interesting things going on that day inside the ship too. There was a talk on the Northern Lights, about how the phenomena arose and how best to photograph it. I was keen to remember the advice and took notes and photos of the PowerPoint presentation. There was also a talk on killer whales, and we were both most surprised to learn that there'd been sightings off the Australian coast.

After our three-course dinner at the set time of 8.15 p.m. for our group, we went back to our cabin for an early night.

The next day, we reached our seventh stop, the first of two that day. It was at Ålesund on Cruise Day 10, 17 September. We were alongside a pier in the middle of Ålesund city centre and within walking distance of most attractions. We disembarked using the gangway for the first time in a while. I walked off using my stick and holding on to the rail. Sue pulled the scooter along and, as she did so, a crew member hopped in and helped her.

It was early in the morning and the sun wasn't yet fully out. We had to make an early start because the ship would leave at 11 a.m. for our next destination.

Ålesund is an art deco town with a small mountain at its edge. The mountain has many steep steps leading to the top. The view from up there was supposed to be terrific and not to be missed. Thilli and Anni were going to walk it. They set off to go up there straight away. I was most impressed. I'd seen the small steep mountain from the ship, and it looked like mountain-goat territory.

Fairly soon after disembarking, we met up with Kerrie and Bob and discussed going up the hill. We thought we'd walk around town first, keeping an eye out for a taxi rank, and then we'd go up the hill together in a taxi.

We walked around looking at the art deco buildings and taking photos. When the sun came out, the reflections in the little harbour were stunning.

We also saw the sinking MS *Nordlys* ship in dock around the other side of the harbour. We'd heard in an earlier ship announcement that one of the twelve Hurtigruten coastal-run ships had got into trouble. It had returned to shore and all the passengers were safe, but the ship was listing at nearly 22° after having taken too much water on board. The authorities were trying to pump it out before the ship rolled over.

We heard later that there'd been a fire in the engine room. Two members of the crew had died and sixteen were injured. It was a sad and dramatic event.

In another dock area, a man and his young son were selling crabs from a boat. The large crabs had been caught only hours before. More photos! Time was passing and it was now only one hour before we were due back on board the ship. It was time to go up the mountain. 'Has anyone seen a taxi?' asked Bob.

'No, none at all,' Sue replied.

'Did anyone notice a sign?' I asked.

'No. What should we do? said Kerrie.

The four of us stood in a car park just off the road where we'd seen a sign indicating a taxi rank. There was no taxi anywhere in sight. I started looking on my phone for a universal taxi number for Norway. Then, one suddenly appeared! It was a station wagon. Fantastic, I thought.

The scooter and the four of us were all quickly inside the taxi and the driver took us up the long steep twisting road to the top of the hill. It took about fifteen minutes to get there. At the top, there was a building with a flat concrete surround. The building, a tourist cafe, was closed because it was the end of the season. There was a good level area to walk around outside the cafe, with a lookout at one end. We all got out and I got on my scooter to go straight to the lookout. We asked the taxi to wait for us.

The view from the lookout was fabulous. I took a photo looking down on the town with its reflections and our moored ship. The photo was as good as, or better, than any postcard, I thought. Looking more closely, I could see two Hurtigruten ships, one on each side of the town. The MS *Fram* was the one that wasn't sinking!

I was so pleased that we'd decided to go up to the lookout later in the morning and not before. With the sun well out by the time we got there, the scene was perfect. After enjoying the view, we bundled back into the cab without much time to spare. Going down the steep winding hill, we listened to the driver talk about his town and the area. We had only about ten minutes up our sleeve by the time we reached the ship.

The views from the ship as we left Ålesund and went out along the fjord were beautiful too. We were sailing in fjords within fjords again, with farmland and brightly coloured houses by the water's edge. Then the low land became mountainous. The edges rose steeply out of the water and waterfalls tumbled down. We were heading for Geirangerfjord.

These fjords in south-western Norway are spectacular. I'd never been to an area of such enormous beauty. Milford Sound in New Zealand is tiny in comparison. There are so many fjords in that area of Norway, and they're interconnected; one turned around into another. Once again, it was hard to follow exactly where we were on the map and, once again, I stopped checking and just looked at the wonderful scenery around me.

I knew we were generally travelling south most of the time. Sometimes we went east into fjords and then twisted our way in all directions before going out west to turn left at the coastline and head south again.

The ship's notes for the day said that Geirangerfjord was 'one of Norway's most visited tourist sites' and that it was 'listed as a UNESCO World Heritage Site, jointly with Nærøyfjord'. There it was, I thought. At last, the name of that fjord had appeared – Nærøyfjord – the name of the smaller fjord associated with the Nutshell. Nærøyfjord was further inland, east and south. Geirangerfjord was bigger, more well-known and it was nearby.

At about 3 p.m., the ship moored in a fjord near a steep cliff. An announcement asked that those going on the hike to Skageflå Farm and on towards Homlong be ready on Deck 2. The farm was among a small number of abandoned farms that had been restored.

The polar circle boats were organised and about twenty people got into two boats, ten people in each. The boats went over to a very small sandy beach with only a couple of metres of level land behind it. The cliffs rose almost vertically from there.

I stood on deck and watched. Sharon joined me. She told me her husband was in the hiking party. 'He's very fit,' she said. 'He goes to the gym a lot, does lots of walking. I wish I could do it.' I remembered Sharon's bad knee.

We stood and watched the people climb up the steep mountain. Some hike, I thought. I took photos of some very rickety-looking wooden walkways around the mountain, with ropes to hold on to. I'm glad it's them and not me, I thought. The closest thing I'd done to that was the walk on our holiday years ago at Lord Howe Island in the Tasman Sea, on the other side of Mt Lidgbird. At the time, I begged Sue not to go any further. She was so close to the edge and it was a long way down the steep cliff. To certain death, I thought. I refused to go any further. I burst into tears. Sue finally agreed and we went back down the side we'd come up using the rope rails.

The group on the mountainside in Norway soon disappeared up into their climb. The boats came back, were loaded up and the ship left to moor near the town of Geiranger for our second stop of the day.

The ship moored in the middle of Geirangerfjord in front of the little town of Geiranger, our eighth stop, on Cruise Day 10. There was a tender boat service to go ashore. We had another excursion booked there, the 'Geiranger Panorama'. We waited for an announcement telling us to be ready. I asked Sharon if she was coming on the trip. 'I'm not confident that I can do it,' she said.

'Sure, you can. I think you can do it. I'll have my walking stick too. Come with us.'

I'd noticed how well Sharon walked with her stick after she'd told me about her knee. It was when we were toasting our far northern position out on the deck on Cruise Day 3. She looked quite stable to me; she got about without too much trouble. But she didn't want to go in case it upset the surgery she'd had.

'I haven't booked,' Sharon said.

'There's still plenty of time before we go. Why not go and try? It'll mostly be sitting on the bus, I think. That should be okay,' I encouraged her.

Sharon went off. She came back not long after, and she'd booked the excursion.

I rode my scooter next to Sue and we all got into the polar circle boat. I wasn't sure if I'd need the scooter or not. The walk from the pier to the bus might be a long way, so even if I just used it for that it would be worthwhile.

There were two buses, one with an English-speaking guide and one with a German-speaking guide.

I'd noticed a steep zigzag road up the mountain on portside as we came to the end of the fjord at Geiranger. That's where we went on the bus. With every turn there was a better and better view. There were farms on the steep sides, with animals grazing. I wondered how they stayed upright. The road closed in winter and the only way out for people living in the area was by boat.

We reached a viewing area on the mountainside and everyone got out, including me. I just used my walking stick and Sue's arm. Sharon got out slowly with her stick and I took a photo of her. It was a nice photo, with a lovely view of Geiranger, our ship moored in the fjord, the snow-dusted mountains and flowers in the foreground. 'If you give me your email address later, I'll send it to you when I get back,' I told her.

I thought maybe that was all the excursion was going to be, but not so. After we all got back into the buses, we went down the mountain, past the pier, and on through the small town of Geiranger. After another viewing-point stop – one not suitable for me because it was far too steep – the bus went inland and towards the snow-topped mountains.

We went past raised lakes, a few houses and one small hotel, all in largely deserted, rugged, rocky countryside. We then went on what we were told was a private road up another very steep mountain. My eyes were wide open as we went close to the edge. We seemed to be going above the clouds. The guide explained how we'd gained access to the road and about the small rocks grouped together now and then not far from the road. 'They are for the trolls,' the guide said.

When we arrived at the top, there was a large flat bitumen area for cars and buses to park. Around the edges were concrete paths and waist-high fences protecting us from a steep fall to the bottom of the mountain.

I got out and the driver opened the compartment in the lower section of the bus to unload my scooter. He and Sue lifted it out. It was very cold and also windy. I hopped on and went over to the concrete paths to check out the views. They were fantastic. I think we could see back to Geirangerfjord. Then it started to snow!

'Quick, let's get some cover over there,' I said, pointing to some new-looking metal buildings. They were along a short path to the edge, and turned out to be the toilets. There was also a very nice-looking disabled toilet with an appropriate sign. It struck me as incongruous, all the way up here, so isolated, and yet here was a brilliant disabled toilet – with a view! I had to take a photo of that. Then I became even colder and hotfooted it back to the bus.

The snow gathered around us; people were laughing and throwing snowballs at each other. It was a bit magical. I wondered if the trolls were watching us.

The buses drove back down the mountain and the guide told us more about the area. It was warm in the bus and we listened keenly. Before too long, we were back at Geiranger and the pier.

While we'd been away up our own mountain, the polar circle boats went over to the other side of the fjord from the pier. They picked up the hiking group and brought them all back to the ship.

Yet another excursion had been going on too. It had taken people overland by bus from one of our ship stops to meet us up again at the next stop. It gave people the opportunity to see further into the countryside and look down into the fjords from above.

I loved seeing the fjords from the ship. I could see so much natural beauty in the mountains and waterfalls all around us. But I might try by land another time, I thought.

We really enjoyed our excursion and we had even more than usual to talk about over dinner that night. After dinner, the ship's crew put on a show for us in the observation lounge. It was our second-last night on the ship and some of the crew members dressed up and sang for us. It was funny seeing them out of uniform, singing and dancing. Every one of the ship's crew had been wonderful to us during the journey.

The ship continued travelling further south during the night.

The next day, Cruise Day 11, the ship wound its way in and out of many more fjords and waterways until it reached a dead end at Olden. We were in Nordfjord, the sixth longest fjord in Norway. That was our ninth stop. I took two photos of our location on the TV screen in our cabin to record where we were. (Photo 3.4.3 and Photo 3.4.4)

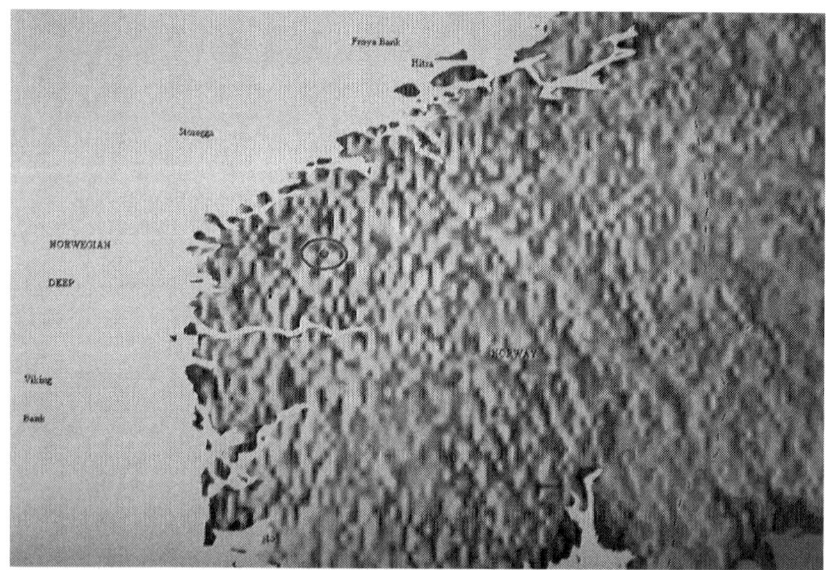

Photo 3.4.3 Ship's position at Olden – Map 1

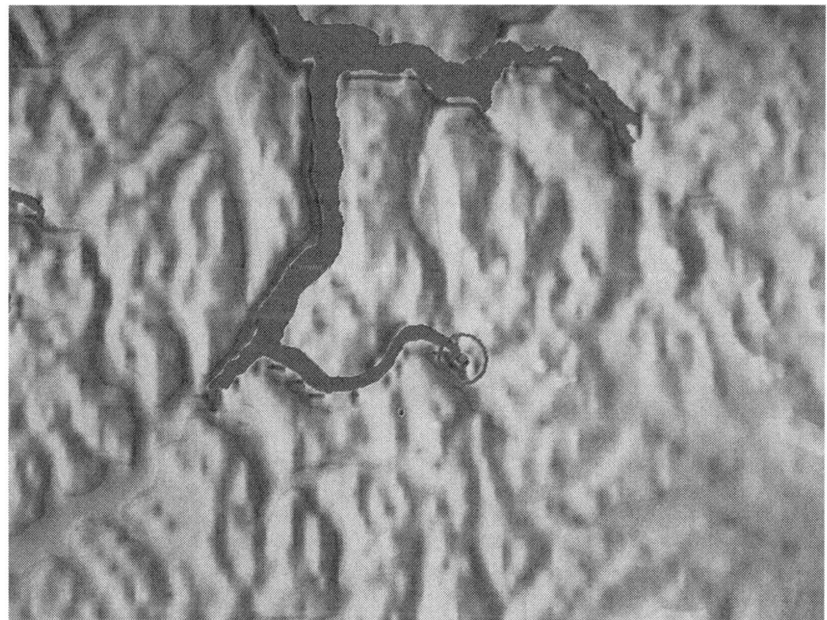

Photo 3.4.4 Ship's position at Olden – Map 2

Thilli had mentioned an old church in Olden that she thought would be worthwhile checking out. We agreed to all go and see it together.

There were many people going out on excursions from Olden that day. One involved walking over a glacier, so I didn't think I'd be able to manage it. We'd only picked out about three extra excursions to do on the second part of the cruise. That was based on what Carolyn told us. She said there was quite a bit to see just by getting off the ship and walking around the town. But only one or two of the places we stopped at ended up being the same as the ones on her Norwegian coastal trip. Her ship took a different route. Most of the places we stopped at were very small, and sometimes there was no town at all. We only learned that as we went along. We'd opted for a walk around Olden.

We met Thilli and Anni on the roadside pier. The gangway was out, so it was easy to disembark. I got off my scooter at the top and walked down with my stick, holding on to the rail. The gradient down was very easy. The tide must be perfect, I thought. Sue rolled the scooter down; it was a bit bumpy for her going over the level beams of wood that ran across the ramp, but she managed all the ups and downs. I waited at the bottom of the gangplank. We put the scooter up and off we went with Thilli and Anni.

The ship was moored against a concreted area beside a bitumen road. It was right at the end of Nordfjord. There was no township of Olden – no shops or anything. Instead, there were a few houses beside the road and some farmhouses sitting on small hills in green, grassy pastures. The views on our right, across the road, were of fjord waters with hills and mountains rolling skywards. We continued on our path on the left side of the road and moved into a valley. The four of us were the only people around.

I noticed some very beautiful flowers along the side of the concrete path and stopped to look at them. Sue didn't know their names. She said she'd forgotten most of the things she'd learned in her horticultural course. That wasn't her main training anyway. She did that course out of interest. Like me, Sue loved science, and she had a bachelor of science degree (but not in botany).

Also beside the path were some poles with large banners flying. They read 'Briksdal Glacier, Jostedal Glacier National Park'. The path finally led to a collection of houses near a small bridge. There was only one main road. We turned left and soon saw the church. Thilli had it marked on her map.

When we reached the little wooden church we saw a sign out the front, impressed in some sort of metal and mounted into stonework. It read:

> OLDEN GAMLE KYRKJE
>
> VIGSLA 1759
>
> KYRKJER PÅ SAME TOMT FRÅ FØR 1308

I took that to mean that some sort of church had been in this location since 1308 and that the current building was from 1759.

That was before Captain Cook came to Australia in 1788, I thought.

The church had two large wooden doors, which were open. Inside, it wasn't like any church that I'd ever seen before. Everything was made of wood. I left my scooter on the thin grass outside and stepped over a wooden board that sat up high at right angles at the entrance. I suppose it was there to keep the snow out.

There was wood everywhere. The floor, the pews, the pictures, the altar, the lectern, the lightshades, the signs – everything was made of wood. There were even antler-shaped woodcarvings to hold the blinds.

The words painted high over the entrance to the altar were '*Gud Signe Fedralandeti*'. I thought part of this must mean 'God bless', and after that was something that I'd look up later. I'd never seen a church like this one. It was simple and childlike, but also seemed to be full of old customs that I had no idea about.

It was a Sunday, and there may have been a service in the church earlier that day. But we were the only people there for most of the time. Then a man and a woman came in, with another younger man talking and explaining what was in the church. They didn't come from our ship. The couple asked some questions with loud American accents that broke the silence. They didn't stay for long, and our peaceful observations and contemplations continued after they left without much talk between us. There were just hushed 'hmms'.

After leaving the old church, we went left again and up the road into the valley, where we could see another church in the distance. Thilli certainly likes churches, I thought. We went past two houses and people came out to look at us. We said hello. They looked at us a little strangely. I thought perhaps people didn't go past these houses very often, or maybe not at that time of year. I thought later that it could have been me they were looking at, and my scooter. Sue stopped briefly and talked with a woman.

The road soon turned into dirt and petered out near the second church. We turned back. When we arrived back at the fjord, there was a wooden bridge to the left and the road went over to the other side of the fjord. The bridge was over a stream, which ran through the valley and gushed down into the fjord. It was an unusually beautiful colour, I thought, a milky blue-green. It was lovely, and the reflections of the old rural houses at the still edges of the stream looked nice too. I stopped and took some photos. I do love reflections! It wasn't that I'd ever been talented in the arts department, but there was nature, being arty right in front of me, and at least I could capture that in a photo.

Not being arty doesn't worry me. I know I have other talents. I believe everyone had some sort of gift for something. But, for some reason, I'll always remember my first attempt at flower decorating. I was in kindergarten or first form at the time, and it was my turn to arrange the flowers in the vase. When I'd finished and stood up to show the class, everyone laughed! Loudly! Arranging flowers to look attractive was obviously not one of my talents. But I could turn out the occasional attractive photo.

After I stopped trying to capture nature and caught up with everyone, we all went back to the ship together.

Later that same day, I ran into Bruce. 'We're just back from the excursion to the glacier,' he said. 'It was very good. We got into a small train on wheels and it took us all the way along the glacier. We could see it quite easily. There wasn't much walking at all. It was wonderful.' He stood with his two long walking poles with those little feet on them.

Oh, I thought, I got that one wrong. Nevertheless, the little church was lovely. The walk and scootering outside in the sun with the flowers, green grass and beautiful waters of the fjord had been a pretty good time. Still, the glacier…

I looked up where that excursion had gone. It went to the Briksdal Glacier. That's what the banners were advertising – trips to Briksdal. I looked up information about the glacier in my *Lonely Planet Norway* and in the ship's information notes. Apparently, people come from all over the world to visit it. The glacier is one of the most accessible and best-known arms of the Jostedal Glacier. It's located at the end of the Oldedalen Valley, about twenty-five kilometres south of the village of Olden. Jostedal is Europe's largest mainland glacier. It looked beautiful.

The excursion list on the ship's noticeboard had two going out that day. They were listed as:

- Briksdal Glacier Walking Tour
- Briksdal Glacier with Troll Cars

That's where everyone was that day – on one of those two tours. It was clear to me by then that I hadn't done a lot of reading about the excursions or about this area of Norway. I was just gliding along and going with the flow. That was enjoyable too.

Perhaps the water of the stream near the little church in Olden was that colour because it came from the glacier, I thought. We had probably been in Oldedalen Valley.

The ship left Olden and went back into Nordfjord to wind its way to the coast. On the way out, we would have one more stop in fjord waters. That was to be at Nordfjordeid, and there was to be an excursion to visit some little ponies there. Sue would like that, I thought. Then, when we were looking at excursion bookings again, I noticed that it was one of the cancelled ones.

We landed at our tenth stop of Nordfjordeid later that day, using the polar circle boats. It was late afternoon and I was feeling a bit tired. In two hours' time, there was going to be a barbeque dinner on deck, for our last night on board the ship. I decided not to go on the landing but to go back to our cabin and rest instead. Sue went out alone.

After resting, I realised that it was about time I did my leg-stretching exercises. I lay on my front on the bed and bent one knee, with the other leg helping it move back a bit. Then I put my hand back to grab my ankle and pulled it down to touch my buttock, holding the position for ten seconds. Then I slowly lowered my leg straight out on the bed again. I repeated the movement with my other leg. I did twenty leg movements in all, ten for each leg. My thigh muscles felt the stretching the most. I can always tell if I haven't done that exercise for a while because my thighs feel stiffer, it's harder to bend and it hurts more. I was supposed to do that exercise three times a week. Sometimes on holiday, I forgot.

Sue came back and we changed for dinner. The weather was good that evening but we still had to rug up to have dinner outside. We met up with Thilli and Anni and enjoyed a great barbeque buffet dinner together. The sunset around us was fantastic.

Anni raced up on to one of the top decks. She'd spotted a photo opportunity. Later, when I saw her photos, I could see why she'd ventured up there. Anni's photo showed lots of people, including those at our table, on the deck with the fjord and mountains in the background and the sun starting to set.

Then there was another photo that she took with the sun setting behind the Norwegian flag that flew out from the ship. It was a beautiful photo, with the sunset and flag positioned perfectly, one behind the other, with water and mountains around them. (Photo 3.4.5)

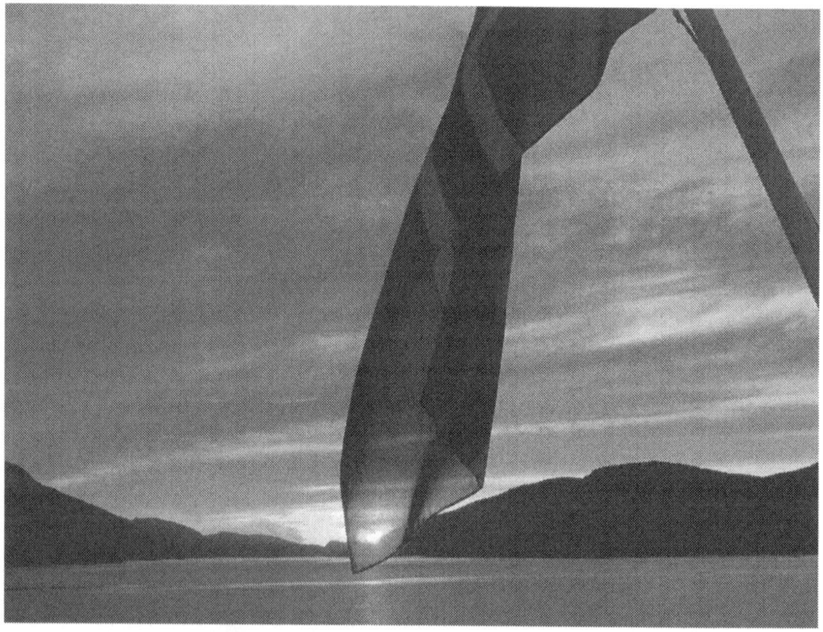

Photo 3.4.5 Anni's sunset photo from our last night

The ship left the fjord at about 8.30 p.m. on Sunday, 18 September. The wonderful barbeque was a very fitting end to the expedition cruise. The name of our cruise was 'Polar Bears, Islands and Fjords'. We had seen them all.

After dinner, Sue and I left the deck to go to our cabin to pack. Tomorrow, we'd be waking up in Bergen. That would be Cruise Day 12, and our eleventh and last stop. We packed our bag and I plugged the scooter in to recharge once more on the ship. And then we went to sleep.

I felt very content. I was full of so many wonderful memories of our Norwegian trip so far. There was more to come, but I didn't want to think about that then.

CHAPTER 5
PEOPLE ON THE SHIP

The first person I met from the cruise was a man whom I sat beside on the flight to Longyearbyen. I think his name was Rolf. He was Norwegian and had worked in the Svalbard decades earlier. He wanted to come back and see what it was like in 2011. He seemed to be a keen photographer, and took many photos from his window seat. I leaned forward to take mine with my superzoom lens. We nodded to each other. I saw him quite a few times after that, taking photos, and we'd nod to each other each time.

Bruce and Helen, who were from Colorado, were both interesting people with whom to pass the time. One day, I found Bruce in the cafe, sitting on his own, and I joined him. Bruce was a professor at the university in their home town. We had an interesting talk about reading. I remember telling him about a movie I'd seen called *The Reader*. There were many aspects to that movie, I thought. To be able to read and write was one thing that struck me as being ever so important. Bruce said he hadn't heard of the movie but he'd keep an eye out for it.

Helen, more than once, referred to us as 'family', and it was true that between us all it was okay to do or say anything. Towards the end of the cruise, Helen told me about her next trip. She was going with a group, without Bruce, to Central Africa – Burkina Faso, Senegal, Mali and other places. She said she'd be doing something in relation to education. I was fascinated to hear about the group's activities.

There was a man named Joe on board who used a walker. His blonde wife appeared to be much younger than him. They both looked Russian but they had broad New York accents. I learned later that Joe was just getting over hip-replacement surgery and that his walker was helping him learn to walk again. His wife seemed devoted to him.

On the first night, we sat with a German group of two couples. One man, Hans, spoke enough English to chat a little over dinner. They'd been on a trip to Antarctica in early summer the year before. They went with Hurtigruten on the same ship we were on now, the MS *Fram*. Hans had taken a video of their trip and turned it into a home movie. He was keen for everyone to see it. The expedition team had scheduled a viewing in one of the lecture theatres.

Hans reminded me, as we passed each other later on the ship, that the show would be on at such-and-such a day and time. Sue and I went to see it. The weather on his trip looked appalling. There were heavy winds, wild seas and sometimes snow on the deck. His wife, when posing for the camera, was almost blown away as she stepped out on to the deck. It was nothing like our trip there. We'd had wonderful weather, with sunshine and blue skies. For us, it had been a warm 10°C on the deck and we'd enjoyed a few barbeque lunches out there. There were two parts to Hans's video, but we only went to one screening. I wanted to remember Antarctica as I'd experienced it.

Then there was Glenda. Glenda was in her late eighties and she was into everything. She signed up for every excursion possible. Glenda had a big, booming, cultured British accent. She was full of life and brimming with energy. On the last night, just before the barbeque began on deck, she was in her swimming costume in the heated outdoor spa pool. I took a photo of her and asked if she'd like me to send it to her. She said, 'Oh no thank you, I've already organised a photo. It's already been taken for me.'

Towards the end of the cruise, Glenda invited us to her very large cabin suite, with its personal balcony, for a drink before dinner. 'You must come and have champagne with me in my suite. There are lovely views through the glass surround, and a balcony off the rear of the ship. It's very private. I always ask for it.' She liked to travel well, I thought.

'Yes, thank you, that would be lovely,' I said. Neither Sue nor I had ever been in a luxury suite on a ship before.

'I'll let you know a suitable night when I can arrange something,' said Glenda.

We joined her for champagne a night or so later. We talked about, or rather we listened to, stories about her life. She'd spent many years looking after her elderly parents and then an invalided husband. 'It's time for me now!' she announced. 'I love travelling and I've not been able to do much of it in the past. And I always try to do it with some luxury.'

I asked where she was going next. Glenda replied, 'Oh, the Gulf of Bothnia. I'm booked on a cruise next month.'

I'd never even heard of the Gulf of Bothnia! I found out exactly where it was as soon as I could. I liked to repeat her words sometimes – 'Oh, the Gulf of Bothnia.' I could still hear her saying it for a long time afterwards. Sue and I thought she was fantastic.

Everyone on the cruise seemed to love travelling and exploring. It was wonderful to be surrounded by people with the same passion.

The two other Australians on the trip, Kerrie and Bob, with whom we chatted and took walks, were good fun too. Bob was a bit slower than Kerrie, so Kerrie walked with Sue, the fast walker. I could control the speed of my scooter to go along beside Bob. My scooter can move up to six or seven kilometres an hour, which is a fast walking speed, but I can also go much slower quite easily. Bob talked about computer systems with me. He said that he used a Linux system to operate his network at home. My IT knowledge didn't extend to that level, and I thought I must look that one up sometime.

Bob and Kerrie were in their seventies and seemed to be experienced travellers. I thought this cruise was not quite adventurous enough for them.

At one stage, the ship moored in a fjord in the south of Norway to wait for an excursion to return. I was on my own on deck, looking at the beautiful scenery around us and taking photos. I suddenly felt like having a cup of tea. I went in to the buffet area, made myself one and sat at a table in the bistro. It was open twenty-four hours a day and you could help yourself to tea, instant coffee and biscuits. It was a pleasant area, with big windows to look out from. I'd often sit there with a cup of tea, feeling very happy.

One day, when I was there, an elderly man, perhaps of Mediterranean descent, approached me. His English wasn't good but it was better than my attempts at any other language.

'Do you play backgammon?' I gathered he asked.

'I've only played once or twice but I'd like to know how to play better,' I replied, nodding my head.

We played a few games of backgammon. He was very good and very fast. He started out being reasonably patient with me, but I could see that I wasn't fast enough for him. I felt a bit of tension grow between us. I don't think I was an interesting enough player for him. In fact, I'm sure I wasn't.

I like those images of Greek islands where the men sit outside cafes and play board games. They know how to play. I thought I should learn to play better sometime. Well, to play the game at all, I realised, after playing with this man. I thanked him and took my leave. He gave me his business card, which showed an address in Tripoli.

Sue and I both went to the bistro a few times for a cuppa. We even made plunger coffee there in the new Bodum travel plunger that we'd bought on sale at a coastal stop. There were a few closing-down sales in towns along the way. It was the end of the tourist season on the Norway coast.

We also learned along the way that many locals in the north of Norway went to Spain in winter. They closed up their homes and businesses and moved away for a whole season. It was at times quite cold outside on our ventures, and it was nice to go back to the warm and cosy bistro. I could understand the idea of moving away from somewhere cold when it became even colder in winter. Melbourne could become very cold in winter too; my Spain was Queensland.

There were some people in the bistro whom I didn't see again anywhere else on the ship. They seemed to prefer that area to any of the other places. There was also another set of people who always made for the big comfy recliner chairs up in the observation lounge, right up close to the big windows.

I also noticed a very large obese man at meal times in the restaurant. He was always enjoying a lot of food, which was set out in front of him by his travelling companion, a small woman who looked as if she was of Asian heritage. She always brought the food to him. Sometimes she sat with him and sometimes she didn't. He was on his own at other times too, writing in a journal. It wasn't until the second-last day, when he came over to help me move a chair, that I spoke with him. He surprised me with how caring and kind he seemed. From a distance, he seemed to be quite aloof and possibly brusque.

I found out that he was a journalist from Copenhagen and he was writing a review of the cruise for a magazine.

I met his travelling partner not long after talking with him. I asked her where she was from. 'I am Danish too,' she said in well-spoken English. 'We both work in Copenhagen. We live together.'

I wished later that I'd spent more time talking with both of them. Something about them interested me.

In the last hour on board the ship, the younger of the two Japanese women to whom Sue and I had spoken was frantically searching for us. 'Oh, there you are!' she said. 'You must have these.' She gave us two little sets of bells on a coloured cord. 'Thank you, it was lovely meeting you,' she said as she rushed off.

'It was nice to meet you too, and thank you for these,' I said. We'd met up with the two of them a few more times after the flu vaccine exchange and didn't have any other differences of opinion. I didn't know what the bells were at the time but I felt her sentiment when she gave them to me. I found out later that it's customary for Japanese people to give a gift to people they meet.

Sue and I had been in the observation lounge only once in the evening, before the final evening's crew performance. On that other night, there was music, drinking and talking, and I found it difficult to have a conversation anywhere in the area. One group seemed to be a little intoxicated, and became loud and unruly. But everyone else seemed to be happy sitting around and enjoying the band. On other nights, there were scheduled events such as ice-carving or vegetable-peeling competitions. We didn't go to them. I didn't meet many people in the lounge on the nights we went.

We usually had dinner late and by the time we were finished we were happy to go straight to our cabin. Sue would write up her diary and I'd go through my photos. We'd also read up on what was happening the next day, or reflect on something that had happened that day.

Sometimes, people tried to help me. Sometimes it worked out well and sometimes it didn't. Help was offered at times when we needed it and at times when we didn't. My reaction to people wanting to help me often depended on how difficult the situation was. And it was always coloured by bad things that had happened in the past.

***

Bad things have happened to every one of my mobility devices. Parts have broken with airline travel and wear and tear, but some other incidents have been the result of people trying to help. There are some broken parts that I can fix myself, but most need a professional technician. Getting something serious fixed usually means a trip to a workshop and a period of time during which I can't use the device. That would be especially disastrous if I'm out of the country on holiday! So Sue and I usually like to look after my mobility devices on our own. It's safer that way, and Sue has learned to ask for help when she needs it.

Once, when I was boarding a ferry in Melbourne to go across Port Phillip Bay to Williamstown, a man grabbed my yellow scooter from us by its tiller, lifted the whole thing up and put it down roughly. He broke the tiller-release cable. The scooter couldn't be moved or collapsed. 'Please leave it alone,' I said. 'We can manage it.' I was very cranky with him.

I was still able to ride the scooter when we got off the ferry, but only by leaning much further forward than I normally did and by holding on to the handlebars on the top of the upright tiller with my arms fully stretched out. I definitely looked odd! It was a bit difficult, and things got even worse when we reached the car. The scooter wouldn't fit inside with the tiller fully up.

My old blue wheelchair had motorised parts that grabbed the tyres and moved the wheels around. More than once, conditions slowed it down, such as when I was going up a hill or across a loose surface. It could sometimes look as if I needed help to go faster, but I didn't; the wheelchair was just going more slowly than it usually did. People would come along and push from behind to make it go faster, forcing the motor and wearing down its parts. 'No, no, no!' I'd call out. 'Please leave it! You're forcing the motor.' Sometimes people listened and sometimes they didn't.

They really were just trying to help, I'd tell myself. They cared. But a whole mix of emotions would run through me when things like this happened. I really wished they'd just ask first. Please, Maureen, try and stay calm, I'd tell myself. This thought would be followed by others: please don't think you know better because… Please don't assume I know nothing because… Please don't take over... Then I'd say to myself again, Maureen, they didn't know, they were just trying to help, for goodness' sake.

There have been other times when helpful people have turned out to be a godsend. Sue and I have been helped out more than once when we were struggling. It was wonderful, then, to be helped.

But I can get really anxious about my mobility equipment. I've always wanted to be independent; to remain independent, I need that equipment so I can get to places and move about when I want to. I feel hopeless without it.

When I travel, I'm especially worried that something will happen and that I'll have to be without a mobility device. It's my lifeline, my connection to the world and to everyone else.

***

Getting around the ship and going on shore with my scooter had been wonderful. There were no problems as a result of people trying to help out on the MS *Fram*. Any help we received had worked out well. Members of the crew sometimes helped Sue with the scooter and that was no problem either. In fact, it was a great help and they looked after the scooter with care.

There were other people on the ship using mobility aids. There was the man from New York with a walker, Sharon with her walking stick, Bruce with his walking poles with funny feet, Glenda with her walking stick seat, and me with my walking stick and my scooter. They all seemed comfortable and at ease with using their devices.

But sometimes people find it difficult to discuss walking aids. 'You won't catch me using one of those things, I'd rather be dead than use a wheelchair.' 'I'm not giving in.' 'I'm afraid I'll get used to it.' 'I don't need one.' 'I'll know when I do need one.' I think I've heard it all. And then they fall.

***

I'll never forget seeing an advertisement for a travel scooter in an MS Society magazine some years ago. I thought it was great, especially that the magazine was for the first time showing its readers what kind of equipment was available. Not only did I think it was great but I also thought it would be a good idea if, in the future, there was information in the magazine to let people know when new ideas and new equipment came out. So I was shocked when I read in the Letters to the Editor section of the next issue a response from a reader that was exactly the opposite of mine. The person was objecting to the picture of the scooter. The letter read something like, 'Not all people with MS are in or will be in wheelchairs or scooters.' They thought the picture and advertisement shouldn't have been included. They seemed very upset by it.

My response, apart from being shocked, was to yell, 'It's okay to be in a wheelchair or scooter!' But I was used to it by then. It was certainly hard in the beginning.

So I do understand people's reluctance a little. I looked around a lot after I bought my first walking stick to see if anyone was looking at me. But that stick made my walking so much easier; it meant my body used less energy and made me feel much more confident. I stopped looking around fairly quickly.

When I used a scooter for the first time, it didn't feel right. It took me a while to find one I liked and to get used to it. But when people become fixed in their opposition to wheelchairs, scooters, walking sticks or walkers, it just doesn't make any sense to me at all. These things are aids to help people; they're not for looks.

Is it pride? Do people think they might look old? Is it about being looked at in a strange way? I can't figure it out. Is it that I've been using my aids for so long that I've forgotten what it was like in the early days?

***

A free CD of the voyage was left in our cabin at the end of the trip. The CD held a lot of information. There were daily programmes, maps, sailed distances, *Fram* history, team photos and also information on the nationalities of people aboard. (Table 3.5.1)

Passengers by Nationality

COUNTRY	NUMBER
Austria	13
Australia	4
Belgium	6
Switzerland	7
Denmark	14
France	9
Japan	2
Philippines	1
Great Britain	24
Norway	26
Sweden	2
USA	24
Germany	80
TOTAL	**212**

Table 3.5.1

When people saw our identification tags with 'AU' on them for our nationality, they thought we were from Austria. They were most surprised to learn that we were from Australia – 'so far away,' they said. I'd do a sort of jumping kangaroo simulation to clarify things and people usually laughed and nodded.

From my observation of the demographics of our fellow passengers, I thought everyone looked over forty years of age. Most would have been over fifty. The age range would have been about forty to eighty-five, and the male/female ratio would have been about fifty-fifty.

Even before I saw the list of passenger numbers by nationality, I thought the group was a good mix. As a group, we all seemed genuinely interested in the areas we visited. The group seemed to be respectful, responsible and caring. They weren't loud, didn't swear and were full of interesting and often intelligent conversation. All their accents were different. Their customs, cultures and ideas were different. I liked to travel with groups like that. They were part of the experience of travelling overseas and being out of Australia.

On a few tours in the past, I'd found that an all-Australian group sometimes didn't work so well for me. I'd felt like I was still in Australia a lot of the time – Australians travelling in one tent and camped together on one side of the global village. I didn't feel as if I was really a part of the wider world that was opening out in front of me.

On these tours, there always seemed to be somebody who was loud, difficult or annoying. Then, I suppose, there are always people like that on whatever tour you're on. If someone is speaking in a different language and being annoying, I suppose I wouldn't know about it. But maybe those all-Australian tours were just the wrong kind for me. That's probably why there are so many different types of tours, to suit many different types of people. And, regardless, some personalities just mix well and others don't. People might find me annoying – going slowly and getting anxious when someone is just trying to help. But for me, there just didn't seem to be enough variety, balance, newness, multiculturalism or worldliness on those particular Australian group tours.

Yet, when it came time to return home, there was sometimes nothing lovelier than to hear an Australian accent when you hadn't heard one for some time. And then to launch into the familiarity that speaking the same language with the same accent brings.

On that CD, there was also a list of the nationalities of the crew members. I thought that was interesting too. (Table 3.5.2)

Crew by Nationality

COUNTRY	NUMBER
Panama	3
Philippines	55
Indonesia	1
India	2
Norway	11
TOTAL	72

Table 3.5.2

There certainly did seem to be mostly Filipino waiters and waitresses in the dining room. They were always happy, and looking to help and please everyone.

Then there was the expedition team. (Table 3.5.3)

Expedition Team by Nationality

COUNTRY	NUMBER
Canada	1
Chile	1
Germany	3
Netherlands	1
Norway	2
Poland	1
USA	1
TOTAL	10

Table 3.5.3

The members of the expedition team were busy working most of the time. They gave talks, prepared reports, investigated conditions when we were going to land, and did many more things. They also seemed to keep to themselves a lot of the time. Or perhaps I was just too shy to approach them.

I did approach one of the expedition team members to talk about how inaccessible the cable-car trip had been, the one that had been advertised as wheelchair-accessible. This particular team member didn't seem to be too concerned, and I was annoyed with him. I thought the information in the notes should be correct so that people would know what to expect. I sat there waiting for him to say something. He finally said he'd look into it.

Mostly, the expedition team was very professional. There were no special instructions for me. The team just handled things as they came up and they handled them well.

We were on the ship from 5 p.m. on Thursday, 8 September to 8 a.m. on Monday, 19 September. For our 'twelve day cruise', that was eleven nights and between ten and eleven full days. It seemed much longer than that.

I didn't talk to anyone on the cruise about the Nutshell trip. I hadn't thought of it for a long time myself. I was having such a fantastic time that there wasn't any opportunity to think about it. Perhaps, in the back of my mind, I thought there wasn't anything I could do about it on the ship anyway. There were so many other things to do. I thought that I'd look into the Nutshell again in Bergen after the cruise. That was our next stop.

CHAPTER 6
BERGEN

The MS *Fram* pulled in early to the port of Bergen. I woke and we were there. 'Quick! Breakfast,' I said. We had to disembark by 8 a.m. All of a sudden, it was a rush.

Up the stairs went Sue, up in the lift for me, to the dining level. We met Thilli and Anni for breakfast at our arranged time of 7.15 a.m.

Towards the end of the meal, some of the other people we'd met on the ship stopped on their way out of the dining room to say goodbye. We all wished each other well. Finally, it was time to say goodbye to Thilli and Anni. There was a lot of hugging and sad looks.

Sue and I headed back to our cabin. Luggage bags and bundles of sheets filled the ship's corridors. The cabin crew were already making up the rooms, stripping the beds and removing rubbish. I noticed that some of the crew doing the cleaning were the same staff from the dining room.

We went to the bathroom and then packed the toothbrushes and grabbed our bags. I rode my scooter up the hall with my small backpack on. Sue rolled the big bag wearing the bigger backpack. When we arrived in the foyer, people were lined up everywhere to disembark. No one was moving yet.

We'd scored seats in a bus that was delivering passengers to two hotels organised by Hurtigruten. I'd booked a different hotel.

I knew it was close to one of the other ones and thought we could walk that short distance. There were other buses transferring people, including Thilli and Anni, to the airport in Bergen.

Thilli and Anni met us in the foyer. It was very crowded. We parked our bags in a corner and went up to the top of the ship and out on to the deck. Together, we looked out on the city of Bergen.

I remembered what Bergen looked like from my map. I'd looked at the map in detail when I was thinking about how we'd get from the ship to the hotel and by what means. I'd originally thought of catching a taxi. But where I'd thought the ship would be berthing wasn't where we were now. We were right in the city, at the old docks. We weren't seven or eight kilometres away from the city centre. The city was right in front of us. Time to figure out the directions later, I thought. Besides, we were going by an organised bus. I'd figure it out on the way.

There was just the four of us on deck. It was quiet. I'd just stopped thinking about directions when Thilli said, 'I will not be going to Australia again.' By this, I thought Thilli meant that she wouldn't be seeing us again.

I said, 'We'll come over here, to Europe, again. We'll send you an email.' We'd exchanged phone numbers as well as postal and email addresses, and checked the spelling of our names the day before.

Anni said, 'It was a lovely trip.' Her English had improved. Unfortunately, my German had not! We all stood there for a little while not saying much. I thought that we were all wishing that we'd had more time to get to know each other.

Thilli soon indicated that it was time they left. There were more hugs, vocal noises, goodbyes and waves. We all left the deck and once inside again we collected our bags. 'One?' asked Anni, who'd just noticed.

'Yes.' Our one luggage bag seemed to intrigue most people. It was easiest for Sue, and we were proud of ourselves for being able to manage with one bag.

We waved to our new German friends as they went down the

stairs. Sue and I went down in the lift and then lined up patiently and waited for our turn to go out down the gangplank to disembark.

Some of the other passengers kindly let me go ahead. I was able to get down the whole way on my scooter. The angle of the gangway was near-level and there were no gaps or blocks going across it. It was a different ramp to the one we'd been using on the cruise – much better, much easier.

Then there were more queues. We found our line for the bus and waited. I could see most of the other passengers who were going to the airport walking past us. Some of them looked quite different. It was interesting. Some of them wore different clothing to what I'd seen them wearing on the ship. They were more dressed up or had more make-up on or something. Some people also had different types of luggage bags to the ones I'd seen before. I always found those kinds of things interesting.

We were soon on the bus, my scooter safely in the lower luggage compartment. It was only a short drive of probably about one to two kilometres. We could have walked and scootered ourselves, I thought. We were in a flat, central area of Bergen. We got off the bus at a big hotel overlooking the harbour, and I scootered a few hundred metres to our hotel, the Augustin. It was raining. Everyone had said that it always rained in Bergen. I'd forgotten about that.

The short ramp into the hotel was at an odd angle and I had to concentrate so as not to fall over. Then we were inside, feeling, and I'm sure looking, like drowned rats. The reception staff were warm and welcoming. The mood inside the hotel foyer area was also friendly. There was a separate lounge area with coffee tables, books, magazines and papers to read. One side was glass, looking out on to the street in a discrete way. I didn't feel I was in a goldfish bowl. It was much more private than that. There was also tea- and coffee-making facilities and a waffle machine. I'd read about that in the hotel information. It said, 'The mix should be freely available at 4 p.m.' for people to make themselves waffles for afternoon tea.

After checking in and looking about the foyer and lounge

areas, we left to go up to our room. The first lift we tried couldn't fit the scooter. It was less than a metre deep with no room to turn sideways. One of the hotel's staff members noticed. 'You should be able to fit in the other lift, further around the corner, over there.' Oh, that's right, I remembered the email. We went a short distance away and, although it was a tight fit, the scooter fitted and we successfully travelled up two floors.

There were many modern paintings on the walls along the corridor and in the room. Similar paintings were in the foyer and lounge areas too. I thought they looked good. The room had a disabled-friendly bathroom and plenty of room to move around. There was also a small lounge suite facing sideways to a television set. 'This all looks good,' I said.

'Yes, it does.' Sue arranged the bag and backpacks in the room. 'I feel like a cup of tea,' she said. We went down to the lounge and made ourselves a cuppa. Then we sat and planned our next move in this new rainy city. It was still too early for a waffle!

It was tempting not to go out. We could see what it was like out there from the cosy lounge. It was still raining, and I still had my wet-weather gear on. I'd worn my wet-weather pants just about every day on the ship. They kept me warm as well as dry. We had three days in Bergen ahead of us. I looked outside, thought for a while and then said, 'Well, it was raining in Oslo and we managed to get out and about.'

'I'm just waiting for you,' said Sue. Off we went. Although we'd just had a cup of tea, we were really hanging out for a good cup of coffee.

I'd read about a good coffee place in Bergen. It was a cafe run by the same family who ran the Augustin where we were staying. When we'd arrived at the hotel earlier, we'd had an enjoyable conversation with the young man at reception. He'd told us about the hotel's history and the family who owned it. He also told us the directions to the cafe. We headed out and went there first.

It was not straightforward getting to that cafe, but we made it. It was in a shopping complex in an old three-storey building on a corner. The cafe was around the corner and off another street, hidden. But oh, was it worth it! They served excellent coffee and the cafe had a nice feel to it. Sue chatted to the barista about where the beans came from and where they were roasted.

As it was still raining, we thought we'd do some indoor things. We looked at some shops and then went to the tourist information office a few blocks away. I had questions about the Nutshell. I still wasn't happy about going out on to the fjord and not being able to get back. I needed to find out more about the bus going back to Flåm.

The man helping us said there were two timetables for the bus, a summer one and a winter one. He checked the timetable for the date that we'd be in Flåm for the Nutshell, 22 September.

'Yes, there looks like there is a bus stopping at Gudvangen at 6.25 p.m. on that day, going to Flåm,' he said.

'What about getting tickets?' I asked.

'You just pay when you get on the bus,' the man explained.

'Good,' I said. I also checked that the ferry times I'd looked up were correct.

'Yes, those are the times. And you can buy tickets for the ferry at the pier on the day.' Excellent. All those connections should work.

I read some of the information in the tourist centre about Bergen. I learned that seven hills and seven fjords surround Bergen and that in the twelfth and thirteenth centuries it had been the capital of Norway. The Hanseatic League of German states was an economically powerful trading group at that time. Their first office was in Bergen at the waterfront in Bryggen. The port was an extremely busy hub then.

While we were in Bergen, we wanted to go and see the home of Edvard Grieg, the Norwegian composer. I enjoy listening to classical music and have heard some of Grieg's works, such as the ones in *Peer Gynt*, a play by that other famous Norwegian, Henrik Ibsen. We also wanted to go to one of the concerts that were held at Grieg's house. There were tours and concert bus trips advertised, but neither of those choices appealed to us as a way of getting there.

I said, 'Well, we can always get a taxi, especially if it's raining.'

Sue asked about getting to Grieg's home by train, tram or public bus. The man at the tourist information counter explained the train system. The nearest station to Grieg's home in Troldhaugen, where the Edvard Grieg Museum was also located, was a station of the same name – Troldhaugen. That seemed easy. 'Let's just get the local public transport and see a bit more of Bergen,' said Sue.

'Okay,' I said, 'but let's see what the weather is like first. We're not going there today.'

Some days later, when the weather looked like it had improved enough, we headed off to Troldhaugen. Getting on and off Bergen's city trains was easy. The entry into the carriages was level with the platform; the gap was small and suitable for my scooter wheels to ride straight over. Sue checked when we had to get off with some of the other passengers.

We got off at the train at Troldhaugen and then realised we didn't know whether to turn left or right. We looked around and saw no one to ask. Then we saw someone disappearing off the platform, way down to the right. We rushed off and asked our question. Yes, that was the way and we were on the right track. There weren't any signs to help us until a few streets away.

As we were walking and scootering along, the clouds started to darken. We'd been lucky so far, with a few hours without rain. The rain stayed away and the walk to Grieg's was lovely. It wound up and down streets, bridges and waterways. I took a few photos and Sue a video or two. The route that we were walking had a nice feeling about it – the autumn trees, the houses, the grass and the occasional stream. I was pleased that we'd come by train.

We went past a cycle path with signs to the city. I said, 'Gee, this might be another way of getting back – along a bicycle route to the city. It might be a nice way to go. I wonder if my battery would last the distance? I suppose we could always charge it at the museum when we get there.' Sue was off videoing and didn't hear me. She was busy taking in a lovely scene.

A parking area with a sign out the front emerged from a wooded area. Cars and buses had to park in a large bitumen area and after that it was pedestrian-only access along a narrow driveway of dirt and gravel. There were no vehicles parked there when we went through. Good, I thought. No crowds.

The slightly muddy driveway went through trees and gardens for about two hundred metres, leading us first to the museum. We continued past the museum to arrive at Grieg's home, which was set on a hill overlooking the waters of a fjord. The whole area had a park-like feeling, with what looked like at least an acre or so of land around the buildings. I left my scooter parked outside and we went into Grieg's home, the Villa. It was where he'd lived in the later years of his life. We saw the original furniture, carpets, paintings and photos that had surrounded him. His Steinway grand piano was still there too. His home seemed simple and quiet, with inspiring views to the fjord through the windows. We were the only two people on the house tour and I really enjoyed hearing about the man and his life.

Troldhaugen, the home of Edvard and Nina Grieg, was built in 1884–85. The waters of Nordåsvannet surrounded it. Grieg had lived and worked there every summer from 1885 until his death in 1907 at the age of sixty-four.

Concerts were held in another building, a small hall near the house called Troldsalen. Inside the concert hall, a grand piano and a small stool sat up on a stage. The back wall of the stage was of floor-to-ceiling glass. Behind the piano, through the glass, were trees and gardens and the waters of the fjord. A small wooden cabin sat close to the water. The whole beautiful scene was like a framed picture. The wooden cabin was where Grieg composed his works, looking out on to the fjord. It was in full view everywhere inside the concert hall.

An attendant gave us a concert programme as we entered. The programme said that Rune Alver would be playing Grieg's piano music that day. The items in the programme were written in four languages. Listed in English, the pieces were:

Once upon a time
Summer's Eve
Puck
    All from Opus 71, and
Solveig's Song, from Opus 55 no 4
Ballade, Opus 24, extracts, and finally
Wedding Day at Troldhaugen, Opus 65 No 6

The concert went for about an hour. We both really enjoyed it. The scene behind was perfect to gaze out at while the music played. I let my mind drift off to the sounds and the feelings coming from that idyllic setting – like a feather floating on a gentle breeze over the water.

We applauded at the end and sat quietly for a few more minutes. Then it started to teem with rain outside. It was the heaviest fall we'd seen in all our time in Norway. We were getting quite used to the idea that it always rained in Bergen! It had been raining very lightly before, when we walked the few kilometres from the train station. But now we had to walk back. I thought and said again, as I often had, that we could always call a taxi. There's no excuse not to go somewhere, I agree, but there's no need to get completely wet if you didn't have to either.

Luckily – what an incredible coincidence! – just before the concert had begun, we'd bumped into Bob and Kerrie from the cruise. They were on a half-day bus tour with only about eight people on it. 'Why not just come back with our group?' said Bob. 'The tour finishes here and we're going back to the Bryggen area in the city. I'll speak with the tour guide. It's too wet for you to go out on your scooter.'

Bob went off to talk to his tour guide and Kerrie stayed with us. The rest of their group, including the guide, had headed down the driveway in the rain to get back into the bus. We waited under cover and I packed my camera safely away while Sue chatted with Kerrie. Bob came back in a little while and said, 'Yes, that's okay. The tour guide spoke with the bus driver and said that if you just gave him a little extra money for his trouble, it would be fine for you to come with us.'

'Great.'

We went off as fast as we could with Kerrie holding an umbrella over my head. There was no time to visit the museum near the entrance and see it as well. We'd left the museum until last because the tour of Grieg's home had been scheduled to start only minutes after we'd arrived. We planned to go back.

In the car park, a large modern bus with plenty of room inside was waiting for us. It had a luggage area on the underside, suitable for my scooter. Sue supervised the driver as he lifted and rolled it in. I climbed up a few steps to get inside the bus and sat down at a window seat.

On the way back into the city, I looked around at the suburbs and views. Sue and I looked at each other and said almost at the same time, 'You just don't get the same feeling for a place on a tour bus.'

The tour guide spoke into a microphone and explained where we were, and told us various facts and figures about Bergen and Norway as the bus sped along the main roads. The population of Bergen was about 250,000. I couldn't take in anything else that the guide told us after that. It was difficult to see outside in the rain and it really was just a means of transport back to the city. We were dry and warm.

'I think we managed that trip well,' Sue said later. 'The train trip and the walk from the station at Troldhaugen were both great. How lucky to bump into Kerrie and Bob and get the bus back too.'

'Yes, amazing! And just at the right time. We could have been drenched.'

'When I was talking with Kerrie,' Sue added, 'she said they'd heard on the news at their hotel that Sam Stosur won the US Open Tennis Championships. It happened while we were on the ship.'

'Really? Wow, that's fantastic!' I said. 'That's her first Grand Slam singles win, isn't it?'

'Yes, it is. There's some hope yet for Australian tennis.'

On another day in Bergen, as soon as the rain stopped and the sun looked like it would break through the clouds, we went over to the old funicular station on the other side of the dock area. The Fløibanen funicular had been modernised and it was wheelchair- and scooter-accessible. Inside the station building, there was a lift that went up to a mezzanine area from where I could ride straight into one of the carriages with a wheelchair sign on it. Access to the other carriages required steps. I took a photo. It was so easy to get inside that funicular; the photo would join my growing collection of examples of accessible public transport.

The views out of the glass windows and ceiling of the funicular were wonderful. We went up a very steep hill; surprisingly, quite a few suburbs of the city were located there. There were stops at many of them. It was mainly the locals who got out, the people of Bergen who were using the funicular that day. It was just another means of public transport to them. It certainly seemed the best way to get up such a steep hill.

The view from the top was terrific too. We were so high up. I could see the MS *Fram* still moored at the dock. I knew it would be there for a few days because Bob and Kerrie were getting back on to it to go on the ship's next expedition voyage – to the Orkney Islands, Scotland, Ireland, finishing in Southampton. From up there, I could also see the rest of the fjord spreading out from Bergen towards the sea.

It was very windy at the top of the hill and I had to hold the rail firmly when I stood up to take photos. We went on a walk and scooter to look around. The restaurant up there was closed for winter. Everything in Norway seemed to be closing down at this time of year. It was the second half of September and I was still surprised at how early things were changing. It was true that some of the places we'd visited on our cruise had been either closed or in the process of closing for winter. But they were much further north. I hadn't realised that parts of Bergen would be closing too.

We went for a walk away from the funicular line. There was more of the hill to climb, but the trails were muddy after the rain.

I didn't get very far. Sue went on and I stopped to look at the forest that was all around me. The pine trees and fir trees at the top of the hill were lovely. There was also a small wooden cabin tucked down in a hollow off the path, so I went a bit further and waited near it. The Norwegians really like wooden cabins, I thought.

When Sue came back from her short walk, she said, 'There's a great view of the other side of Bergen around that corner.' She pointed to her left. 'The path has some gravel on it, but you should be okay.' I scootered along the path and there were good views, quite different to those in the other direction. There was no water, just the suburbs of Bergen. There were a lot of three- and four-storey apartment buildings and one eight-storey one. The scene wasn't pretty but it was interesting. The apartment blocks were grey and vaguely reminded me of public housing blocks, or perhaps, once again, something with a Soviet influence.

We went back to the funicular stop and into an adjacent souvenir shop. I bought a couple of postcards and looked about at the souvenirs. The weather was changing outside. We went back down in the funicular, looking out through the glass panelling above our heads and around us. The rain became heavier; it completely surrounded us and blocked the views of the fjord. We waited for a while at the base station under cover, but the rain wasn't clearing. We left the station and headed home to the hotel as fast as we could with our hoods on. It was time to re-charge my scooter battery – and ourselves – before heading out again.

We went out to visit new places every day. We covered most of the city, including the university at the top of a hill, as well as going to the dock, up more hills and also to parks on the flat ground, surrounded by art galleries. I began to feel really connected to the place.

At the end of one day, just as we were going back to the hotel, my left foot started to go numb. I knew I'd been sitting on my scooter for most of the day and I was keen to get back to our hotel room.

That feeling in my left foot happens if I haven't been moving my legs or feet much. Sometimes, it happens even if I *have* been moving them. The numbness usually lasts for about thirty minutes, but it can go on for a few hours. It's a funny feeling. It feels like a *nnyy … nnyy …* a buzzing feeling. Sometimes it feels as if my whole foot is swelling up and, occasionally, that does happen.

I have to stand and push my toes down, or sit and try to lift them back up, or reach down with my hands and move my foot. After a while, it can feel like it's burning; but it was different to the other burning patches I sometimes got in odd places on my arms, legs or back. I find moving around and putting my feet up helps.

Sometimes the odd feelings are not in my feet. They can be anywhere. Pins and needles, numb patches or prickly feelings – I feel as if I have to move the area about to stop the sensation. That doesn't really make much difference, but elevating my legs does help a bit.

On that day in Bergen, it was time for a rest in bed anyway. I thought I must also remember to do my exercises at least two or three times a week, even if I was on holiday! That might help too.

On another day, I rang Mum one morning, when it would be early evening back in Australia. 'Hi Mum, just ringing to let you know that we're in Bergen and having a great time. How are you going?'

'Oh, it's lovely to hear from you, love. I've been following you on the timetable you sent me. I thought you must be there by now. Do they still have those old houses down on the water?'

'Yes.' I told her about our trip and some of the things we'd seen. I asked her how she was and what she'd been doing.

'Oh, a bit of this and a bit of that,' she said.

'How's your back? Are the pills working?'

'It's all right in general. Oh, I caught up with Pat the other day and…'

When I was satisfied that she seemed to be managing all right I said, 'Well, we'll be going out soon to do a few more things. It's morning over here.'

'Thanks for ringing, love, and keep having a wonderful time.'

'Okay. Bye, Mum, bye.'

One late afternoon, when we were returning to the Augustin, we both felt like a nice glass of wine. I had my eye on a special wine bar in the hotel. It was a wine cave that was many years old. The family who owned the hotel had only discovered the cave when they purchased the building next door so they could expand. It was a fascinating story. When the renovations were taking place, they found a cellar built as interconnecting caves under the building. It hadn't been opened for decades.

I'd read about the wine bar in a few different places. I saw it as a side note in one of my guidebooks, in one of Sue's wine magazines and in an in-flight magazine on the way over. The place had won awards in the *Wine Spectator* magazine for its range and quality. I'd definitely noted that place in my mind.

Late afternoon was a perfect time to go into the wine cave, and we just happened to find ourselves there one day. Somehow, I managed to walk in and around with the help of my walking stick and Sue's arm. I left my scooter near the hotel reception.

There were a few people at the small bar when we went in. A woman was serving. She told us we could have a glass at the bar or we could go through into the caves and sit at a table. We thought we'd decide which wine we wanted first and then venture in to a table.

We asked what was available. I think the young woman was looking at us a little strangely, perhaps trying to ascertain what language we were speaking, what accent we were using or what knowledge of wine we might have. Perhaps people didn't ask what was available. I wasn't sure.

'My name is Christina,' she said.

We introduced ourselves. I let Sue start the wine discussion. She was always much better at that. I loved listening to her. 'I think I'd like something along the lines of a dry Riesling, something that is … and …,' said Sue.

Christina replied, speaking beautiful English. She spoke about a whole variety of European wines that we could choose. Christina spoke of many types that I'd never heard of. I happily let Sue chat on and choose hers. Then it was my turn. 'I'd like something like a Pinot gris or a Soave,' I said.

'I have a nice Chablis that I have just opened if you would like to try it,' said Christina.

'Oh yes, thank you,' I said after looking at Sue for a subtle indication from her to let me know if I should say yes or no. Christina poured tasting samples of our choices into our glasses and handed them to us. I still didn't understand the name of Sue's. I tasted mine and said, 'That's lovely, yes, thank you, a glass of that would be nice. Where is it from?' There was a brief silence, then Christina said, 'From Chablis.'

'Oh yes, of course,' I said. I'd forgotten that Chablis was French and from Chablis. I like to think I was really asking which vineyard it was from. But that's an Australian wine question and probably didn't mean the same thing in France. I felt a bit silly, but laughed at myself afterwards. I thought it would be a good story to tell. I laughed more at myself later when I realised that, sure, Chablis was a wine region, but the grape variety was Chardonnay. It didn't taste anything like Australian Chardonnay; it was much drier and less fruity.

'If you go in and find a table, I will bring your glasses in to you,' said Christina. She added, 'Be careful of your heads, the doorways are very low.'

We went further inside. The walls were white, like in whitewashed Greek houses. Red leather covered the chairs and they looked great against the walls. The tables were white too, and there were brown tiles on the floor. There were multiple rounded rooms and each room led to another. They were all different sizes and there were glass lights hanging on the walls. The light was low. My camera definitely needed its flash. I couldn't see a person in a photo without using it. We took turns taking each other's photos and then sat down at a table to enjoy our wine. We seemed to be the only people there.

After a while, we heard some voices. I remembered reading

about a restaurant near the cellar that had also received an excellent write-up. Further through the cellar, there was supposed to be a connection into it. But we stayed where we were. I thought the hum of the restaurant was a pleasant background noise that added to the ambience.

It was so nice to just sit and enjoy the wine. Sue and I talked about our day and what we'd seen. We talked about the trip so far, friends back home and the people we'd met. The Nutshell was still ahead of us, but I'd stopped thinking about it ages ago and we didn't talk about it then either.

We chatted and relaxed in the wine cave for about an hour before going back into the hotel again. We decided not to go to the restaurant for dinner. Sue had already bought a few things at the supermarket.

The next day, we went back down to the dock area to explore it more. We went for a walk around the other side of the harbour, to the famous area of Bryggen. It was another UNESCO site – Mum's 'old houses down on the water'. The colourful wooden-clad houses, each a few stories high, looked great. They were originally used as both warehouses and living quarters. Some were slanting with age. The Bryggens Museum, built over the original settlement, showed some of the eight-hundred-year-old original foundations. We wandered around and I took a few photos.

In the back streets, we wandered into the grounds of the Leprosy Museum. It was closed; a sign said it was open only from May to August. The museum was located inside an old wooden building that was rather institutional-looking. I thought it might have once been a hospital. Then the penny dropped – Hansen's disease. Armauer Hansen was Norwegian, and he discovered the leprosy bacillus in the 1800s. I read later that Hansen made his discovery in Bergen in 1873. The old building is one of three leprosy hospitals in Bergen. It's the oldest, and is called St George's Hospital. It housed leprosy research archives.

We left the area and walked back to the hotel through the fish markets. The market area had only one tent up that day. Flat canvas covered its top but the sides were open. I remembered seeing similar tents in Carolyn's postcard, the one she'd sent in June, three months earlier. The picture on the postcard was of a busy and colourful fish market in Bergen. Mum's 'old houses' were in the background too. The postcard had a marker on it that read 'In the Trollfjord, MS *Midnatsol*'.

Carolyn must have bought the postcard in Bergen before she started her coastal cruise north and before she boarded the ship. Then she must have written it while on board and posted it later when they were further north in Trollfjord. The Bergen fish market scene looked a busy one in the postcard, unlike now. It was closing down for winter.

We looked at the seafood displayed for sale. There were fresh red crabs, packed salmon and what looked like short fat prawns.

When we arrived back at the hotel, it was just before 4 p.m. That was an accident, of course! Ingredients and a mixture in a bowl had been freshly prepared and had just arrived. Sue was soon cooking the most wonderful waffles without much hesitation!

There was a small boy sitting alone across the hotel lounge room. He was about seven years old. I'd noticed that a woman, whom I'd assumed to be his mother, had left him there while she went into a lecture room a doorway away. I said to Sue, 'Why don't you go and ask him if he'd like a waffle?'

Sue went over to the little boy and bent over gently. Half turning and pointing to the waffle machine, she asked him, 'Would you like a waffle?' He got up quickly and followed Sue to the kitchenette bench area. The two of them made the waffle together. Within a few minutes, he was happily carrying off a plate with a nice thick waffle topped with syrup on it. He sat down quietly and tucked in.

Even I had a waffle. Even Sue had a waffle. I had strawberry jam on mine and Sue had maple syrup. It was nice!

We enjoyed Bergen. We became used to the rain that fell every day. Everyone else was out in it too, with their hoods pulled up over their rain-proof jackets.

One day I saw a woman on a large mobility scooter, wearing a rain-proof covering which reached from the top of her head down to the top of her scooter wheels. She was all in black. The way she looked disturbed me. It was strange. There was just part of her face poking out of a large black object moving along, crossing the street with everyone else. I hadn't seen anything like it before. That event reminded me of how people had looked at me strangely in the past.

***

I suppose it's human nature to look at things more intently if they're new. But I don't like it when people stare at someone with a disability, especially if that someone is me.

One of the hardest things in the early days, I found, was appearing in public using a four-wheel walker. The worst place was at the swimming pool. Everyone seemed to look up at once as soon as I came through the gate. It made me feel as if I was strange. I just had to swallow my pride and make my way over to the handrails leading into the pool. I hadn't thought anyone was looking at me when I used my first walking stick in that shopping centre years ago, but, here, at the swimming pool, everyone was staring.

Once I got over to the handrails, I sat on a nearby sunbed. I was wearing my swimming costume under my clothes so I took off my top. I also took off the sandals on my feet with their Velcro flaps. I left them on the sunbed and went over to the pool using my walker. I wound my beach towel around the handle and seat of my walker. I left the brake on, and parked it next to the handrail. I wanted my towel close by as soon as I got out of the pool. I put my goggles on over my eyes and down the steps I went, holding on to the rail to get into the water. When I was in deep enough, I swam away. I thought I swam freestyle well and that would make everyone stop looking. I soon forgot the looks and just did my laps.

Freestyle was easy. That's what they called it when I was learning to swim as a child, or the 'Australian crawl'. I mostly swam over-arm;

that's why I found it so easy. The leg exercises that followed were more difficult. I love swimming and, selfishly, I enjoy it the most when I'm the only one in the pool.

That woman in Bergen, on her large scooter and cloaked in black, was moving with the crowd as she crossed at the pedestrian crossing. No one seemed to be looking at her or disturbed by her presence. I didn't stare, but I certainly noticed her. She was different. Maybe I was just different too, when I entered the swimming pool area that time. Maybe the people around the pool hadn't seen anyone using a walker go swimming before. Maybe they were just curious. Maybe I didn't look old enough to be using a walker. Who knows?

With time, I felt better and I continued to use the pool with the help of my walker. I suppose it was about overcoming my pride and not worrying about being seen. I wanted to use the swimming pool and the best and most practical way for me to get there and manage my towel and goggles was with my walker. I just had to deal with it.

***

I went off on my scooter and no one seemed to be looking at me riding along in Bergen. Perhaps they were, but being on my scooter didn't worry me any more.

Later that day, I felt a burning patch on the underside of my right arm when we were back in our hotel room. 'Sue, would you please just have a look at the underside of my right arm? It feels as if I've burnt it on something, but I can't think what or how. I wasn't near the waffle machine.'

Sue looked and looked again. 'I can't see anything.'

'Oh, that's right, I keep forgetting. It's just the MS and those odd feelings I get. Don't worry, I'll think of something else.' Sometimes this burning feeling lasts for hours or days. I find it best to distract myself by doing or thinking of something else.

While we were in Norway, and especially Bergen, I noticed the different cars that were about. I hadn't seen a lot of them in Australia. I kept thinking about accessible cars and ones with a low loading lip for Sue to put the scooter in easily. I took photos of some of them, so I could recall what they looked like for future car buying.

We were in Bergen for three days and three nights. It seemed much longer than that, as with most periods of time on the trip so far. Somehow, the way I register time when I'm travelling is different to how I feel it pass when I'm at home. Is that part of the attraction?

On our last day, in the late afternoon, we were walking and scooting back to the hotel past some shops when I saw a sign advertising reduced prices for thermal underwear. I thought of Mum straight away. I always try to bring her back a present. She hated the cold weather, and, as she became older, her aversion seemed to get worse.

When we all went to Antarctica, I borrowed some thermals for her from a friend. But she might like some of her own to wear around the house in winter, I thought. The shop had a bright pink set, fifty per cent wool and fifty per cent polypropylene. I thought she'd love the colour, and it was a good mix. So I chose a size 14 top and bottom for her.

'They don't look big enough,' said Sue.

'They're size 14, which should be all right. They'll stretch,' I replied.

'Are you sure about that? Maybe you should ask?'

'They'll be fine, I'm sure. They have the same sizes as us here, don't they?'

I carried the thermals around the shop while I looked at a few other things. I love outdoor-gear shops and sporting shops. Sue found something she was interested in and asked the shop attendant about the size for herself. 'Is it for a child?' asked the shop assistant.

'No, it's for me,' said Sue. 'Why? Are these children's sizes?'

'All this area is for children. The adult sizes are over there.' I looked at the hot pink thermals in my hand. They came from the children's area.

'Is this size 14 for children too?' I asked.

'Yes.'

'Oh, I see. Do you have this colour in an adult women's size?' I asked hopefully.

'Yes, we have small, medium and large sizes for adults. Over there.' I went over and found several hot pink sets in all sizes.

'What do you think of this one, Sue? Mum has been getting smaller. Large or medium?'

'I think a medium should be fine.'

'Yes, I think so too.'

I bought the hot pink medium thermal underwear set. Gee, I thought, imagine if I'd bought the size 14. Mum would've had a lot of trouble squeezing into a child's underwear! It certainly paid to ask. Yes, Sue had been right. I should have asked earlier.

We left the shop; it was raining again. I hid my new treasure under my black Gore-Tex jacket and pulled the hood up over my head.

Not far from the outdoor-gear shop was a small supermarket. We went in there to get some more provisions for dinner. We bought fish, cheese and salad, and put them in the scooter's backpack. We still had some wine in the fridge to finish with it.

The hotel was only a little way away from the pedestrian-only shopping strip where the supermarket was. We went out into the open area and it was just about deserted. Most of the shops had closed and there were a few street lights coming on. After going out and along the shopping area for a short way, we went down the footpath of a side road. The hotel was on the corner to our left. There was just one steep part at an odd angle on the footpath, so I got off the scooter for a few metres in case it tipped over.

Back at the hotel, I had a rest while Sue watched some golf on the TV. There always seemed to be golf being played somewhere in the world. We had dinner in our room and then packed. We watched a little more television for the weather, Sue wrote in her diary and I deleted some unwanted photos. Then we went to bed.

It was our last night in Bergen and time to move on the next day. We planned to walk to the station the next morning and catch the train to start the Nutshell and see into its kernel.

CHAPTER 7
THE NUTSHELL

The next morning, 22 September, we walked to Bergen Station with plenty of time to spare. It was a grand old building in the middle of the city.

We'd done a trial run several days before on one of our walks. We wanted to check where the accessible entry was and where the platforms were. I also wanted to pick up our tickets well ahead of departure. The disabled entry was around to one side of the old bluestone station building, with no signs at the front to indicate where it was. It took a little while to find the wheelchair-accessible way. I was pleased we'd worked that one out well before time. It was a concrete ramp and I thought few things could go wrong with that.

Inside the station, we found the correct platform, with clear signs to help. I sat on my scooter behind the rope across the entrance to Platform 2 and waited for the train, minding our luggage. I enjoyed looking around the old station while Sue went off to take a few videos. I took a photo of a highly decorated clock up on a wall, with the words '*Velkommen til* Bergen' written above it. The clock had '*Bergens*' on one side of it and '*Tidende*' on the other, advertising one of Norway's newspapers. I thought taking that photo would make a good start to the next section of my travel photos.

I was the first in the line. We wanted to be up at the front of the queue. Although we'd booked seats, we wanted to get on the carriage early to find enough space for our bag and the scooter.

It was the 10.28 a.m. train. The ticket read 'NSB Regiontog 602 towards Oslo S'. Once the guard let the rope down, we went through and found Carriage 446 easily. Sue walked with the bag and I scootered. When we arrived at the carriage door, a lot of people had already moved past us and boarded the train. I got off my scooter and helped Sue to fold it down. Then I used my walking stick and the handrail to get on. Two Norwegian girls in their early twenties spotted us and jumped up to help.

Once in, I stood in the luggage storage area and held on to a metal post. Sue put the bag on first and then the scooter, with help from the girls. They looked around and said, 'Where are all the men?!' We all laughed.

'Girl power,' one of us said. Those girls did look very fit too.

Our bag was stored with the other baggage that was already there. Sue left the scooter folded down on the floor at the bottom of the luggage shelves and tucked it under a little bit. Everything fitted well.

We thanked the girls. They spoke perfect English. Sue chatted to them briefly and they said they'd not been to Australia yet. We encouraged them to travel there one day and then found our seats and settled down.

The train climbed mountains heading east. There were a few towns along the way but mostly it was empty countryside with a few wooden huts. At the beginning of the trip, I could see fjords in the distance and rivers near the train line. The scene then became mountainous. We soon went across a series of plateaus high in the mountains. One of the plateaus – the Hardangervidda plateau, sits above the tree line and has been described as 'bleak' and 'treeless'. I didn't think it was quite that bad.

On the train, we each had a hard-boiled egg and a bread roll for lunch. We'd packed them to take with us before we left the hotel. After just under two hours, at 12.20 p.m., we arrived at Myrdal. The two Norwegian girls came over to help us off and we thanked them again. They got back on the train to continue on their journey. I thought it was fantastic of them to help us, and they treated the scooter so carefully.

At Myrdal, there was one small train station. There was no town or village that I could see, just mountains. The platform and change of trains was as easy as Carolyn and Ron had said it would be. We just got off the train and walked across the platform to the other side. It was all level, with no steps or stairs. The total distance would have been less than eight metres.

We waited at Myrdal for what the ticket said was the 1.27 p.m. 'Flåmsbana 1857 towards Flåm'. The train arrived almost straight away; it was almost an hour early.

The train was a lovely shiny green, with white writing that read 'Flåmsbana'. In grey was written '20 km long' and in smaller white writing, '*Grandiosa naturaleza*'. It was the famous Flåm Line.

We had plenty of time to board and find seats where the windows were open. There was only one step to get up into the carriage, with a useful handrail, and it was all level inside. There were about six carriages and we could choose any one we wanted. There were no reserved seats allowed on that train. Carolyn had told us that the best seats for taking photographs were the ones where you could open the window. Some windows were fixed glass while others could be opened up or down. She'd also recommended going down the Flåm Line on the right-hand side, the eastern side of the train.

Once in the carriage, we read the information on a video screen explaining the building of the Flåm Line and other interesting facts. I also had time while we were waiting to read some of the brochures that I'd collected. 'Welcome to a trip on the Flåm Railway. An incredible train journey... Nowhere in the world is there an adhesion-type railway ... with a steeper climb... Almost 80% of the railway line has a gradient of 55%.' The twenty-kilometre Flåm Line was an engineering wonder. It had opened in 1940 and climbed 864 metres through twenty tunnels. It was 'one of the world's most attractive and spectacular railway lines'. I'd heard so much about this journey and, after all the planning, I was finally on it.

The train was old but well-appointed. There weren't many people on it. It was the end of the travelling season in that part of Norway too. The train eventually left Myrdal as scheduled and descended into the valley of Flåmsdalen.

The whole journey took one hour, but that time seemed to go so fast. The few people in the carriage were dashing from one side to the other to see the views and take photos. I was happy to sit still on one side of the carriage because I knew we'd be coming back this way and I could sit on the other side then.

Along the way, there were waterfalls, farms, tunnels and zigzag roads on the sides of steep mountains. These roads looked like they were composed of several Zs stacked on top of each other. The valley was made by glaciers millions of years ago. There were nine scheduled stops at small stations between Myrdal and Flåm. The whole trip was wonderful, and I loved the views from the train even though it was a dull day.

We arrived at the last stop of Flåm at 2.25 p.m., and we got off the train without any trouble.

Flåm, at the bottom of the line, is a very small town that sits on the Aurlandsfjord. It has a population of about five hundred people. Its location is spectacular. The water is out in front with mountains rising up around it. I looked back and saw there was an enormous mountain behind the town, where we'd just been on the Flåm Line. That was already one part of the Nutshell that I'd done, and my scooter hadn't been a problem at all.

There wasn't much to see on the ground at Flåm. Once again, almost everything had closed down for the season. I could imagine, though, in full summer, people hiring kayaks, canoes or boats, riding bikes and hiking around the area. The sky might have been brighter then too, I suppose. Now, it was closed in. In fact, most of the days since we'd left the cruise had been dull and rainy with grey skies. Closed in all the time, and not good for taking colourful scenic photos. But I was there.

Flåm Station was less than a hundred metres away from the

Flåmsbrygga Hotel. The ground was level, even and well-surfaced. We passed the ferry terminal office on the way to the hotel, at about twenty metres from the station. There it all was – easy to ride on and easy to get to.

We arrived at the Flåmsbrygga Hotel. It looked a little like the pictures on their website but it wasn't really the A-frame shape that I'd thought it would be. It was more rectangular and longer with a sort of an 'A' at each end. We went down to the entry.

The woman at reception greeted us warmly and said she was expecting us. She took us to our room via a lift at the end of a corridor. When we reached the room, she showed us around and then told us that someone had come there for us a little while ago. The person had asked for a shower chair or stool for me to use. The woman said they didn't have a specific disability stool but she pointed to a small, low, plastic stool in case that might be of help.

Of course, I thought. Carolyn had been to the hotel to check the room months before and had rung me. She knew I had a shower chair at home. She must have asked for one for me.

***

I'd acquired a shower chair some years earlier, in late 2007. Some people in our apartment block gave it to me. Tom and Elaine had been clearing out items after Elaine's uncle had died. I ran into them one day in the car park. They had a walker, a shower seat and an over-the-toilet seat. They asked me if I'd like them. Elaine said, 'I hope you don't mind us asking, but we thought you might want some of these things. I don't mean that you're disabled or anything.'

I said, 'Yes, thank you, that's very nice of you. I'd like the shower seat and the over-the-toilet seat, please.'

'All right, that's good. We didn't think you'd really need this walker, but we'll find a home for it.'

I didn't think I needed the walker then. I was using a walking stick outdoors to help me for short distances, and nothing indoors. I could use the over-the-toilet seat to help me get up more easily, and the shower chair would be good for shaving my legs, I thought. I didn't need it for showering. The seats were a matching white pair and were of good quality too.

Not long after that shower chair came home with me, I really did need it for more than just leg shaving. In March 2008, I had an exacerbation of my MS. I'd just returned from the Antarctic trip and ended up in Epworth Hospital. I thought I might have caught some sort of exotic bug that would account for my extreme fatigue, weakness and walking difficulties, and also for feeling hot. My eyelid muscles were so weak that I couldn't open my eyes for long. The paramedic asked me if I was blind because I spoke with my eyes closed.

When I got home from hospital, I needed to sit in the shower chair when I was having a shower. That was the first time in my life I'd done it. I couldn't stand up in the shower long enough to wash myself.

After a few months, I recovered a fair amount and could stand in the shower for longer periods. In the meantime, I'd had two sets of handrails installed in the shower and they really helped. The chair was still there for a while in case I became tired while standing.

Then I started Tysabri and my MS improved enough over the year that followed for me to feel stronger and more confident standing in the shower again. I didn't need the chair, and I just used the handrails to help me move around. When I'm travelling and using showers with no rails, I can still stand most of the time and just use the wall or screen to steady me.

The one thing from Elaine and Tom that I knocked back was the walker. But that was also something that I ended up needing soon after, and I still use one.

***

When I was in Flåm, in the hotel room with the stool in front of me, many more thoughts flashed through my mind: I must thank Carolyn again for checking the room and asking for something for me to sit on in the shower. Gee, Carolyn was so thoughtful. She was probably streets ahead of me in that department too! I also needed to remember to let her know that I didn't really need a shower chair any more. I was again just using the one at home for shaving my legs. I knew too, in the back of my mind, that I might need it again in the future. But I was okay in Flåm.

I thanked the woman from the hotel reception for the stool. It was in a corner of the room, next to the bathroom, ready to use. The shower was a great walk-in one. It was very nice, with a modern tiled wall running down one side and an opening to walk through and turn right. I thought that the solid walls would be good to lean on a little, if I really needed to, or just to touch. I took photos of the shower. I liked it. I didn't need the stool and left it in the corner.

We'd been travelling for four hours by the time we reached the Flåmsbrygga Hotel. We sat in the comfy chairs in our room and looked out at our lovely balcony. The balcony had its own tables and chairs. Carolyn had taken a photo of that balcony and sent it to us. The view out beyond the tables and chairs was lovely too. We could look out on to the fjord and the ferries passing by.

As I was looking out, it started to rain and the view became obscured with a grey mist. It had rained a lot on this trip, so the rain itself wasn't surprising. But the mist was new. Everything changed very quickly and it became the worst day, weather-wise, since we'd arrived in Norway. Oh dear! Not today! It was the day for doing the Nutshell!

Would we go out on to the Nærøyfjord after all? I said to Sue, 'Look, the trip down the Flåm Line was just lovely. It was a nice train trip from Bergen too.'

'But it's been a full day for you. We can just rest here if you like. We've done pretty well so far. *You've* done well. We've seen some wonderful fjords already,' was Sue's reply.

'It really seems a shame not to go,' I started again. 'Do you think we'd see much in this weather? It's misty, the wind is blowing really strongly and the rain is horizontal!' I reminded Sue (and myself) that Carolyn had said, 'The best way to see the views is out on deck, high up on the ferry, up some stairs. Inside, you can't see much at all.' Maybe I wouldn't get to see much on the ferry trip, anyway, in that weather.

'It's not time to leave yet. We have plenty of time. We can just sit here, see what happens and see how we feel after another five or ten minutes,' said Sue.

I felt less pressure to go out in that awful weather on my scooter, and relaxed a little. I settled down. Then I started to think again.

'It seems a shame. This fjord is supposed to be different to the others. It's the smallest, narrowest one, with the most waterfalls.' I added, 'I'm not even sure the bus will be running to bring us back. The fellow in the tourist office in Bergen said one thing and the fellow in Oslo said another. It seems like the end of the season and all the timetables are changing. What if we go and we can't get back?'

'There must be some way, though. Don't worry about that, we'll manage,' Sue said. 'But do you want to go out in this?'

I thought again and said, 'It might stop soon. What if, as soon as the ferry takes off, the weather improves and we're just sitting here? We'll kick ourselves.'

'Well, we really can't go walking around here, anyway,' said Sue. 'Let's go. You've managed the rain elsewhere. Let's just cover up and go.'

I still had my water-resistant clothing on anyway. I grabbed my camera, and off we went. Down the lift and out on to the paved area to the ferry terminal office. We had to buy the tickets there. That was the one ticket I'd looked at purchasing so many times and hadn't. Sue lined up and asked for two one-way tickets on the next (3.10 p.m.) ferry to Gudvangen. We were going out into the UNESCO-listed Nærøyfjord.

The ferry terminal office was just a Fjord1 ticket counter within a building. There was a tourist office, some fast-food outlets and a souvenir shop. There wasn't much inside, but there were quite a few visitors there. We waited there because we had plenty of time before the ferry left.

Then an announcement came from the ferry outside that all passengers going to Gudvangen should now board as it was leaving!

The time didn't seem to be quite right but we moved quickly to where everyone was getting on.

I was on my scooter; the way for everyone to get on to the ferry was along a wide metal ramp that had been lowered from the rear of the ferry as it pulled in. It looked the same as the one in Carolyn's photo. The metal ramp was lowered on to a concrete loading ramp. It looked as if a small motor vehicle could have been loaded that way.

On to the ferry we went – me scootering and Sue walking ahead, checking the terrain. We handed over our tickets and the attendant explained that I could leave my scooter on the ferry deck under cover, or I could take it inside on to the lower deck. There was a bit of a step-over though, he told us, on the deck separating the outside and inside of the ferry.

We were soon inside. I got off the scooter and Sue rolled and lifted it over the rise. I think the step-over stopped water getting inside. I sat on one of the seats in the wide passageway.

I looked at my ticket. The ticket read, 'Flåm *kai*–Gudvangen *kai*'. I thought my understanding of *kai* was correct – going from pier to pier or quay to quay. But I'd been wrong about the time. It left at 2.56 p.m. not 3.10 p.m. That was fourteen minutes earlier. We'd made it, though. We were on the ferry, rain and all. I kept that ticket. (Photo 3.7.1)

Fjord Fylkesbaatane AS
ORG.Nr: NO976630855MVA
TLF. +47 55907070
fylkesbaatane@fjord1.no

Operator nr. 119106 22.09.11 14:56
Kvitt. 1006020010957 Kasse 2

Flåm kai - Gudvangen kai

2 Vaksen 530,00

TOTAL 530,00

*** Kontant: 530,00
*** Kort...: 0,00
*** Tilbake: 0,00

Type	Brutto	Mva-%	Mva	Netto
0	530,00	8,00	39,26	490,74

God tur
Velkommen igjen
Kan berre refunderast
i lag med billett

Photo 3.7.1 Ferry ticket – Flåm to Gudvangen

I checked out the scene. Back on the scooter, I went down a passageway with glass panels on the right (starboard) side of the ferry. I could see straight out but not up – that is, the houses in the little village of Flåm but not the surrounding mountains.

There was a lounge area to the left with a glass divider between it and the passageway. There were two easy entrances to the lounge and the glass divider gave some protection from the wind that came down the passageway when the door was open. I thought that area might be all right. Then I saw that everyone else had gone further down the passageway towards the front of the boat.

At the front (forward) end of the ferry, there were three flights of metal stairs. The best view was apparently at the very top, as we'd been told. Sue went ahead to investigate. 'Yes, that's where everyone went. They're sitting on plastic seats, which were stacked up all around up there.'

'Oh, okay.'

'There's very little cover out there. There's just a small awning with room for about ten people,' Sue told me. A good forty people would have boarded.

The rain had stopped. I left my scooter at the bottom and ventured up one of the flights of stairs using the handrail and my walking stick. There were some long wooden benches at that first level and I could see out better, so I sat there. At least I could take photos from that position, I thought. Photos from inside wouldn't be worth taking, as Carolyn had said.

The ferry soon set off. The sky was grey and the mist was clearing a bit. The rain was intermittent, light and just bearable. I had my orange lens-cleaning cloth handy, to use every now and then, before and after taking photos. I took photos of Flåm as we left and of Aurland as went past it, along the Aurlandsfjord. Then we went into the larger Sognefjord. Another Fjord1 ferry (similar to ours) passed us, with 'Gudvangen' written on it. Behind the ferry, I could see waterfalls and a few houses on green grass. (Photo 3.7.2)

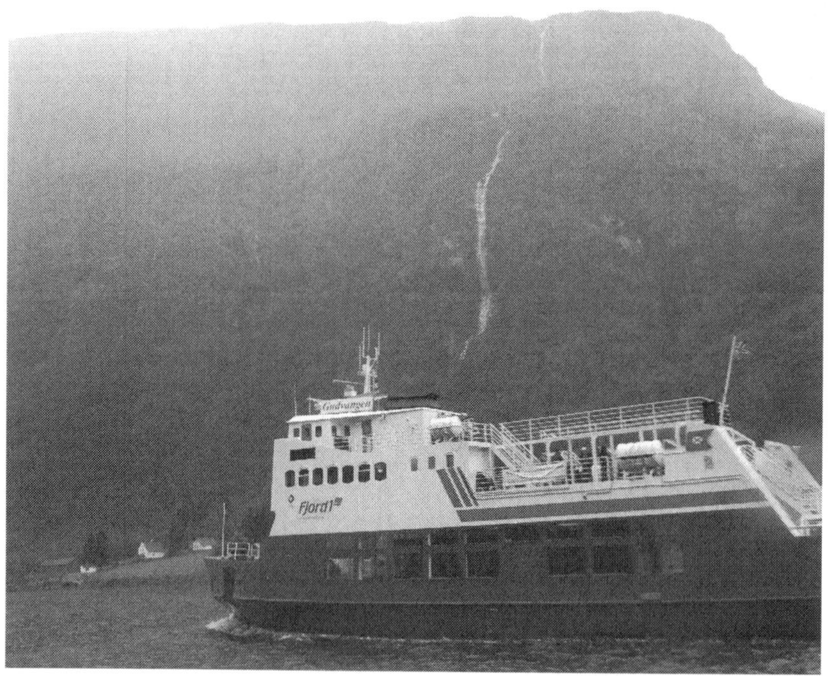

Photo 3.7.2 Another ferry in Sognefjord, passes us when doing the Nutshell

When our ferry took a left turn into a very narrow fjord with high mountains and waterfalls everywhere, I knew we must be in the Nærøyfjord. I was there at last!

I went down the stairs and stood outside at the back of the boat. It seemed to be a better view that way. There were less parts of the ferry in the way. It was a little more sheltered too. The sky was grey and getting darker again, but the scenery was wonderful. As I watched waterfall after waterfall I stopped taking photos. The next one was just one more wonderful waterfall! I just looked at them. The photos on my screen all looked too dark anyway.

Sue was taking video shots. She captured different things to me. I loved watching her videos after we arrived home from a holiday. There was always something funny, or a scene that I hadn't noticed along the way.

Gudvangen was coming up. I could see a few buildings in the

distance. At just after 5 p.m., it was already getting very dark. There was a jetty, one large round building and a few houses. It wasn't really a village or town as I'd expected. We arrived at 5.20 p.m. as per the original schedule, despite the fact that the ferry had left fourteen minutes early. We had time to find out about the bus and look at a souvenir shop.

Most people from the ferry went over to a parking area over on the right, a few hundred metres away. It looked a bit like an open bus stop. There were two old buses parked there. They must be buses to Voss, I thought. As people boarded, I saw that there were steep steps up and no panels outside to indicate baggage storage areas underneath. If I had chosen that part of the route, Sue would have had to drag the scooter up and hope to park it upright in a spare seat. Not impossible, but I'd given up on that bus a long time ago anyway. I was just looking out of interest.

Then I thought about the bus that we needed to catch. From where did it leave? Where did we have to go? Did it come over to that bus stop in the car park? I'd have to ask.

The only public area to go to was the souvenir shop. We went in; at least it provided shelter from the intermittent rain, and it was warm. After a quick look around, I went up to the counter. 'Could you please tell me where we go to catch the bus to Flåm?'

'Up the road, on to the E160, oh, about a hundred metres or so, I suppose,' the shopkeeper told us.

'Where up the road?'

'Just go straight out of here and up the road. You can't miss it.'

'Not just over there where those other buses are?'

'No, it's just a little way up the road.'

It was raining again and getting much darker. We walked out and saw a road leading into the area. I looked around and noticed the rooftops of some of the houses for the first time. They had grass growing on the top and I remembered Mum's postcard of twenty-seven years ago again.

The road ended where the ferry had stopped. Gudvangen was at the end of the Nærøyfjord. Therefore, the road out must be on that road there, I thought. Off we went. As I scootered and Sue walked in the light rain, we saw only a few houses along the way. We were the only ones on the road, and there was no footpath. A single car came past at some stage. The few houses about looked deserted.

It seemed as if we went along for one or two kilometres before we reached another significant road, at a T-intersection. It was not a hundred metres – it felt so much further than that. The road where we ended up looked like a minor highway. A few cars and trucks were racing along in both directions every now and then. Which way do we go? Left or right? Where was the bus stop? There was no structure or booth or covered area that looked like a bus stop. We saw a woman across the road. She looked like she was of Indian descent, about twenty to thirty years old and she had a backpack. She was on our left.

Meantime, a young man came along the road behind us and an older couple came towards him from the right. The young man said, 'Which way to Bergen?'

Bergen! We left there hours ago. We didn't want to go back. Anyway, I didn't think this was the road to Bergen. I thought it was the road to Voss. The couple said they thought Bergen was to the right.

We were waiting on the left corner, off the road, to avoid being splashed by water flying from under the car and truck wheels that sped along past us. Sue went for a walk up to the left to take some videos of the area and came back. Then the Indian woman came over. 'I've looked at the timetable over there,' she said. 'The bus to Flåm is coming soon.'

Yes, I thought, that must be the 6.25 p.m. one that I'd heard about. But where will it stop?

The Indian woman, reading my mind, said, 'Let's go over there in a couple of minutes and wait. It might come early.' That was to the left. They drive on the right-hand side of the road in Norway.

Sue hadn't said a lot, but she was right beside me. We started chatting with the Indian woman while we waited. She was an architect, she said, and in Norway for a conference on environmental design. This was a side trip. I'm not sure how she got there. Maybe she'd come down from Voss. She was doing her own version of the Nutshell. I took a photo of her with the mountains and what I thought was the bus timetable sign in the background.

The older couple had joined us by now, and we all crossed the road together to wait for the bus. We'd agreed that we were going to Flåm by bus and this was the direction and the stop. There was barely enough room for me to sit on my scooter off the road. My scooter is only forty-five centimetres wide, but there wasn't much room there. A metal guardrail formed a barrier to prevent vehicles from going into the low bushland. I took a photo of the bus timetable on a short metal post near the guardrail. It was difficult to read and it was still raining. The print was small but I wanted a memento of the place. (Photo 3.7.3)

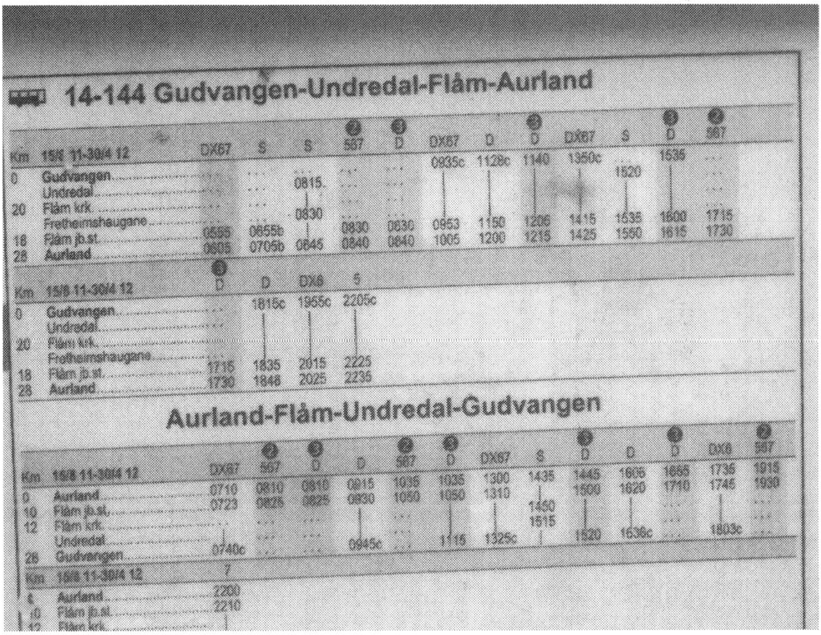

Photo 3.7.3 Bus timetable – Gudvangen to Flåm

A big modern bus soon came along just before 6.25 p.m. A hinged panel opened on the lower part on the side of the bus. The man from the couple helped Sue roll and lift my scooter in. I climbed a few steps and sat in a low single front seat. Perfect. Sue wasn't far behind me. I thanked the man for helping as he went past to find his own seat. The Indian woman paid our bus fares and we paid her back. She told me that I received a discount for being 'disabled'.

The driver of the bus then just sat there, waiting. The bus wasn't moving. I thought perhaps he was waiting a few more minutes for the time to pass so that it was exactly 6.25 p.m. before he drove off. I was still a bit confused.

I had a look at the timetable photo that I'd just taken. I enlarged it so I could read it better. From my reading, the timetable seemed to say that the bus was due there at 6.15 p.m. If that were true, we would probably have missed it! Perhaps, I thought, the bus we're on is the 6.15 p.m. bus and it's late. But then why wait there until 6.25 p.m.? Sue was seated several seats behind me so I couldn't talk with her. Oh dear, you worry too much, I told myself. We were on the bus and that's all that mattered!

The bus did leave shortly after that. Then I saw it – the tunnel through the mountain. That was it! That was the one I'd seen on Carolyn's map. We'd be back at the hotel in Flåm soon.

The tunnel went on and on. I'm not sure how many kilometres it was, but we weren't going slowly and it still took at least ten minutes before we were out of it. I checked the distance on my map. It looked about ten kilometres long. Later, I read that Gudvanga Tunnel is 11.4 kilometres long.

After this ride through the tunnel, lit with lights that seemed to be everywhere, we were suddenly there. I could see Flåm Station a stone's throw away. Wow!

We got off the bus at Flåm, near the station. We said our thanks and goodbyes. It had become truly dark by then. Nothing was open. We offered to walk the Indian woman to her hostel but she said she'd be okay. We went back to our room at the hotel and flopped.

We'd done it – the kernel in the Nutshell. Well, almost. All except that bus trip to Voss. But we'd stood at the base of the mountains and looked up and all around the area for a while. That possibly counted for that part of the kernel.

I sent an email message to Carolyn to thank her for suggesting the hotel room, telling her that it was lovely, and letting her know that we'd just done our kernel of the Nutshell trip.

I think we had some Jarlsberg cheese, bread rolls, crackers and beer for dinner in our room that night. Nothing else was open and we didn't feel like going out anyway. What a day it'd been. I'd done it!

The next day, 23 September, we boarded the morning train in Flåm to do that part of the Nutshell again, in the opposite direction, to make our way home.

It was the 11 a.m. train and the ticket read 'Flåmsbana 1854 towards Myrdal'. A Japanese tour group lined up and got on the train in another carriage. The video screen at the far end of our carriage explained the story of the Flåm Line to us again. Words on the screen showed each segment of the journey in English, German and Japanese.

Then the train left the station at Flåm and we ascended from the fjord at the bottom to the mountains at the top. We sat on the other side of the carriage this time, once again on seats with windows that could be opened. I took lots of photos and Sue used her video camera. The scenery was lovely again, and it looked different going in the opposite direction. There was also more sunlight falling into the valleys and on to the fields. Much better for photos.

It was only yesterday that we'd come down, but it seemed much longer ago than that. John was right, the Flåm is marvellous! And it was marvellous that I was able to do it twice.

We reached Myrdal at 11.59 a.m. I got off first and Sue followed with the bag. Then she got back on to get the scooter down the step. A Japanese woman saw Sue and quickly spoke in Japanese to the man she was with. It sounded as if she'd ordered him to get in and help right away. That's exactly what he did, and the scooter was soon at my feet ready to be set up again on the platform.

That station was the famously unknown one that I'd fretted about so much – Myrdal, where we had to change trains. It had turned out to be so easy yesterday, walking just a few metres from one side to the other side of the same platform, that I didn't feel anxious at all.

We waited to catch the city express train running from Bergen to Oslo. It was to arrive and leave at 12.25 p.m. I thought again that this was the station where Carolyn, with her group, and Ron and Sandra, had changed trains. I recalled once again the photos that they'd taken and emailed to me.

There weren't many people waiting at Myrdal. After a while, we started chatting with four American men on holiday together. They were old friends and caught up once a year on some sort of a trip. They seemed to be in their late fifties. They got along well, and there was lots of laughter.

I looked out at the platform and the tracks. I had my orientation right, I thought. Bergen was to my right, the west. That was where we arrived from yesterday. Oslo was to my left, east.

The Japanese group got on the next train coming in from the left and going to the right, to Bergen. I'm not sure when the penny dropped or who realised it, but suddenly the four American men and the two of us grasped the fact that the train going to Oslo wasn't coming in to either side of the platform that we were on! There were two tracks in front of us and another platform on the other side of them. That other platform had no walkway over to it, no overpass. There was no bridge over the tracks to get to the other side! *That* was the platform where the train to Oslo was going to stop and it would come in from the right to go to the left.

We all realised that we had to get down from this platform using a small ladder at the edge, go across the tracks (where flat metal sheets with small holes lay over them) and climb up the small ladder on the other side. We *had* to get to the other platform.

The only problem was that we couldn't get across the tracks until the train to Bergen had gone! Our train would be coming soon.

We couldn't miss it. We were flying home tomorrow. There was no time to waste but we couldn't move straight away. But we started to get ready. This was a situation that we had to deal with, and fast, whenever the time for action came.

'Well, we're all going to have fun, aren't we?' said one of the American fellows.

Finally, the train to Bergen moved away to the right. The train to Oslo was coming towards us in the distance, also from the right. The four men lifted up our bag, the scooter, their bags and bits of me, and carried us all across the tracks. Sue, with her bad knee, was in among it all. In no time, we were all on the other platform and our train pulled in.

The four men helped us on, stored the luggage and scooter away and then saw us to our seats. They then had to find their own carriage. The train took off. It was so good of them. We thanked them many times as they left us. We were all safely away on the correct train going in the correct direction.

The Nutshell with the kernel side trip turned out to be very memorable indeed! What a station Myrdal was, after all. No one will believe me, I thought. Getting down and across those tracks, then getting up the other side – the scooter, Sue, the luggage and me! Wait till I tell Mum.

I couldn't really relax on the train until I'd thought through what had just happened and why. And then it hit me. Of course! Carolyn was travelling *from* Oslo *to* Bergen and got off at Myrdal to go down the Flåm Line. Ron and Sandra had come up from their ship on the Flåm Line and then travelled from Myrdal *to* Bergen. They got on at Myrdal. None of them had caught the train going in the opposite direction from Myrdal to Oslo. That was probably why the train came in to a different platform to the one they'd been on and photographed for me.

But, *we* came in to Myrdal yesterday on a city express train *from* Bergen going *to* Oslo. When we got off at Myrdal, it was only a few steps across the same platform to get on to the Flåm Line.

Yesterday, the train had stopped on the other side of the platform from where we were waiting, not across the tracks. Why didn't the train we were on now, stop there again?

Well, it just didn't, that's all. The advice from Carolyn, Ron and Sandra wasn't necessarily wrong. The train just came through and stopped at the other platform. Was there a sign back at Myrdal to indicate at which platform the train would stop? Did I check? I didn't recall checking. I just assumed. I expected the train to come in right in front of me. That was wrong.

However, after all of that, it didn't matter in the end. It really was a bit of fun and everyone laughed very loudly when it was all over.

And we were soon high up in the mountains in the central southern area of Norway, going on to the final link in our trip.

CHAPTER 8

OSLO AGAIN, AND HOME

I sat on the train and looked out at the views. Tomorrow, we'd be flying home. It somehow seemed a long time away and I didn't give it much thought. It was the middle of the day and we had the south-easterly section of the line from Bergen to Oslo to travel over yet.

It was at the end of the first month of autumn in Norway – 23 September. There was a lot of snow and ice on the ground. It wasn't very populated out here. The few houses I saw were made of wood and were either situated on their own small lake, or in a group of five or six, also beside a lake.

The train was due to arrive in Oslo at 5.32 p.m., taking five hours to get there. It was supposed to be a very scenic trip, so I spent most of the time keenly looking out of my window, ready to experience it all and take photos whenever I fancied.

At Finse, the first stop, there was an unusual sight. Mountain bikes were lined up, ready for hire, but the wheels were covered in snow. There were a lot of bikes – five lines, with twenty to thirty in each line. They weren't going anywhere soon. I took a few photos. The lines, and lines within the lines, made an interesting attempt at an arty photograph, I thought.

Finse was on a lake, and it looked like a small holiday resort. There was an advertising sign at the station. In child-like writing, it read:

Winter at Finse
Skisailing
Dogsledding
Cross+country skiing
Relaxed and genuine mountain hotel
Check out the hotel and activities at [website] and find your next winter adventures.

There were a lot of other activities in the area as well. Finse, at an altitude of 1,222 metres, was the base for one of Norway's steepest mountain bike rides. Apparently, the bike route included riding from Finse down to Flåm, with stunning scenery and steep hairpin bends along the way. The station at Finse was the Norwegian railway system's highest point and it had no road access. And the glacier nearby - the Hardangerjøkulen glacier, appeared in scenes shot for the Star Wars movie *The Empire Strikes Back*.

After leaving the snow-covered mountains around Finse, we descended on to a plateau with a tundra-like landscape. Once again, we were on the Hardangervidda Plateau, in a large national park. The plateau was the same one we'd travelled across yesterday, on our way from Bergen to Myrdal around the other side of the mountains. It extended across a large part of that area of Norway. When we were heading into Myrdal, we were on the more mountainous western side of Hardangervidda Plateau. We were travelling further east now, and it was flatter, colder and more Arctic looking. The plateau has been described strikingly as 'desolate and beautiful, otherworldly'.

The Hardangervidda Plateau was immense, covering about ten thousand square kilometres. One third of that was included in the Hardangervidda National Park, Norway's largest national park. There were many walking trails and public huts in that wide-open space.

I didn't see any of the herds of wild reindeer that were mentioned in the travel brochures. The largest herd in Norway, of about ten thousand reindeer, was supposed to be located there. I looked out among the mountains, boulders, lakes, rivers and bogs as we crossed the plateau, but I didn't see any kind of animal.

The next hours passed quickly. I stopped taking photos because the afternoon sun was coming directly into my window. The photos I'd taken earlier were blurred. The train was travelling faster than I could take still photos. All that my photos revealed were blurred trees, not the scenic views in between them. I'd read that the Trans-Siberian Railway journey across Russia could be a lot like that – a lot of fir trees out of train windows. But I'd still love to travel across it one day.

After the plateau, there were more lakes, some small towns, pastureland and forests. I sat back in my seat, tucked my camera away and just looked out to enjoy what was there.

When we reached Drammen, I felt we were on the outskirts of Oslo. It was an industrial port as well as the original home of the potato alcohol, aquavit. It was also the start of the old Royal Road back to Bergen. At Drammen Station, I saw the Flytoget train that went to Oslo Airport. Drammen must be a business or commuter centre. We're close to Oslo and our final destination, I thought.

We passed through residential areas after that and headed into Norway's capital city of Oslo once again.

At Oslo Central Station, as we were getting off, the four American men who'd helped us at Myrdal greeted us at our carriage door. One of them said, 'We thought you might like a hand at this end too.'

'Oh, that's so lovely of you!' said Sue.

I had the biggest smile on my face. 'Thank you!'

They all helped and soon the scooter, our bags and ourselves were all safely on the station platform. We wished them well, thanked them immensely and waved them goodbye.

We were at ground level and I could see the city around us. Our Flytoget line was supposed to be underground. When we'd got on and off the Flytoget train before, we'd been at a different station. On the first day of our trip, we'd passed through the Central Station stop, before getting off at the Nationaltheatret stop. Later, we'd caught the Flytoget from Nationaltheatret to go to the airport and fly to Longyearbyen. We hadn't caught the Flytoget train from Oslo Central Station before.

Remembering that experience in Oslo with the faulty lift, I wanted to check out the new territory before we left the station. Even though things didn't work out exactly as we'd planned the last time, I thought I'd feel better if we knew the way. I wanted to see exactly where we were going to catch the Flytoget to the airport the next day.

There were a few different levels at Oslo Central Station, but it didn't take long to work out where to go. There were lifts and travelators (instead of escalators) in obvious places. The accessible routes were well sign-posted and everything seemed to be in working order.

The travelators were flat and much better than escalators for wheelchairs and scooters, as long as the brakes on the devices were on. At the train station, the travelators were on an incline and, with my scooter's automatic electric brake system, I knew I shouldn't roll down. I tested one to check. It worked well. While we were down a level, we saw a supermarket and bought some food for dinner that night.

After satisfying ourselves about where we had to be the next morning, we went up to the top level and left the station on the side of the city where the opera house was. We simply walked out of the train station's automatic sliding doors on to a twenty-metre length of footpath and into a car park next to the Thon Hotel Opera. I'd almost forgotten how close it was.

We checked in to the hotel. It had been a longish day and it was starting to get dark. The lights of the opera house were coming on and I was feeling tired. Our room looked tiny. I could hardly get the scooter inside to charge it. When I checked the bathroom, the shower was over the bath. I rang reception and they said that all the rooms had showers over baths. I hadn't checked with the hotel about the showers before booking. I just looked at the accessibility notes on its website. They indicated that the hotel was fully accessible. Well, the route and path were. Perhaps I should have asked for a disabled-access room, if there was one. I thought that in future I must remember to check what 'accessible' really meant in the advertising.

It was the end of the day, I was tired, I was frustrated and I started to cry. The tears just came out and rolled down my face. I couldn't help it.

***

Sometimes, tears do just come like that. Sometimes, there doesn't even seem to be a reason. I can't control it. It's called emotional lability; being emotionally labile is another aspect of my MS.

When I was admitted to hospital once, the paramedics took me there with my eyes closed as I wept. I couldn't stop crying even as the doctor took my history. Heaven knows what he thought.

At first, I didn't understand why emotional lability would be a feature of MS. The only logical thing I could think of was that it must be related to one or more of the many lesions in my brain. I was really shocked when I read the findings of the first MRI of my brain and cervical spine. The first line of the report said, 'Within the brain there are multiple, at least 30, foci of T2 hypersensitivity,' and 'In the cervical cord ... there are at least 10.' Then the summary of the report said, 'typical for primary demyelination.' I was shocked that I had so many lesions.

I've had more MRI scans since then and I know the disease has progressed. One or two of those lesions must tickle my emotional lability spot, I suppose.

***

I was disappointed about the shower, but bursting into uncontrollable tears was definitely excessive! I just sat there, crying.

'I think you should have a rest. Lie down for a while,' said Sue.

'Yes, okay, I will.'

After a rest, I did feel better. I thought, well, it's only for one night. I'll just have to manage.

That was the only five-star hotel that we stayed at in Norway and it turned out to be the worst place for me. Luckily, it was right at the end of our trip. That day was also the end of the Nutshell trip, at least all the parts of it that I could do. I knew I'd never forget it.

The wonderfully comfortable hotel beds made up for the shower issue and I slept very well that night. I'm sure I dreamt of what my map of the whole trip – Oslo to Oslo – would look like. (Photo 3.8.1)

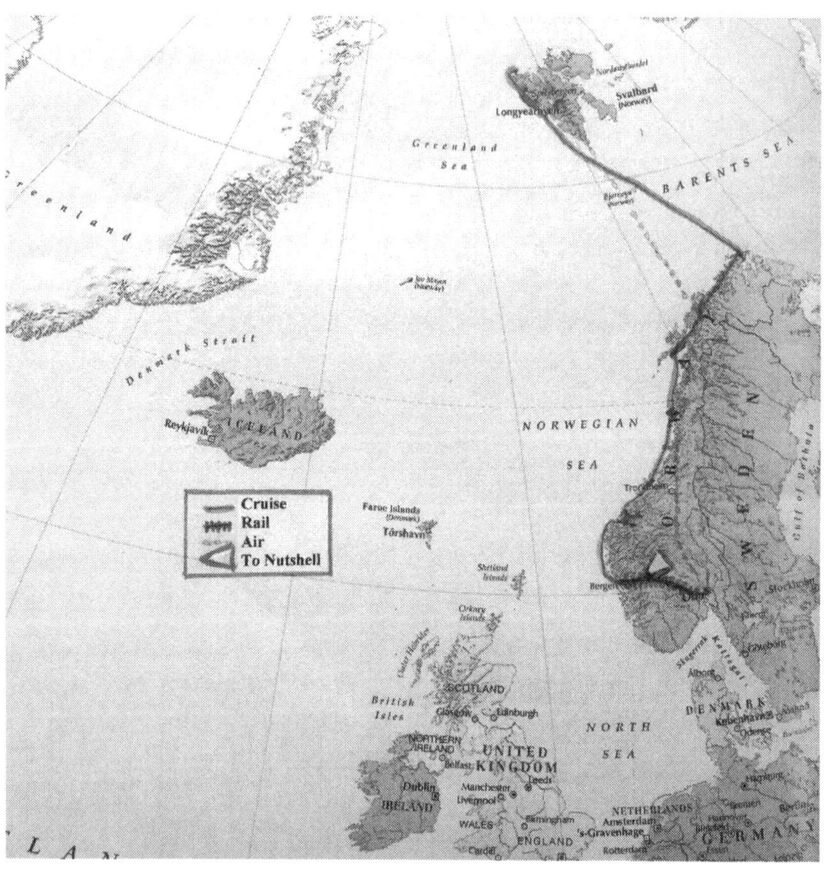

Photo 3.8.1 Map of the trip – Oslo to Oslo

The next morning, Saturday, 24 September, we left the hotel and went the short distance to Oslo Central Station. With our pre-purchased tickets and knowledge of the route, off we went to catch the Flytoget fast train to the airport. The lifts worked and so did the travelators. We were on our way without any problems at all.

Soon after we arrived on the platform, a Flytoget attendant came up to us. We'd met other attendants before but usually in the train, not on the platform. They had all been very pleasant. This one was even better. She said 'Come down to the last carriage and you can wheel straight in. That's the special carriage for bicycles and people with wheelchairs.'

'Do we leave the scooter down there?' I asked.

'You can if you want to, there is plenty of room. But there are seats down there too, if you want to sit on them. Come with me and I'll show you.'

Well, I had sort of heard about the last carriage, but I hadn't really understood. No one had suggested we use it before. Down we went and got into the last carriage of the train without any problems there either. I just wheeled in, parked and got up holding Sue's arm. I used my walking stick to get to a seat. Getting off was just as easy. That was the easiest train trip of all.

When I was doing my planning before the trip and reading the Norwegian State Railways website for booking instructions, it stated that wheelchairs had to be secured at all four points with the person sitting in the chair. But I didn't want to sit on my scooter. The train seat would be more comfortable. The fifty-minute trip to the airport would probably have been all right on the scooter, but not the three- and five-hour journeys from Bergen. Also, to book a wheelchair place, you had to telephone when the office was open. I didn't think I could easily explain what I wanted over the phone. So, I didn't telephone and I didn't book a wheelchair place before leaving Australia.

All we had to do that day was arrive on the station platform and a train attendant took us to the last carriage without a problem. All those worries at home about phoning, I thought.

Then I thought again. This was the Flytoget. It was a different kind of train to the others and was run by a different company. The instructions I'd looked at online were not for this train. Also, we'd caught the Flytoget before and no one had approached us. Oh well, I thought, it'd all worked out in the end.

After fifty minutes, we were at the airport train station. We went out through a ticket gate and into a lift. We went up two levels and there was the airport departure terminal. We booked in at the Thai Airways counter. Once again, I rode my scooter to the departure-gate lounge.

I sat and once again watched airport staff moving about on their large push scooters, delivering and transporting goods. I looked more closely that second time. The person riding had one leg on a wide platform base with wheels. The other leg was moving along the floor pushing the scooter. There was a small basket at the back to carry items. A tall T-shaped steering device came up from the one front wheel and there was also one large wheel at the back. It really was like a child's scooter, only much larger. I thought that it was no wonder people had trouble understanding what I meant sometimes when I said I used a scooter.

When it was time to board, the airport staff took us first. We went along the air bridge to the aircraft door. I got up, did my part of the scooter-collapsing job and Sue did the rest. An aircraft handler took the scooter down the steps to load it into the baggage area. Sue and I boarded the plane just as the rest of the passengers were coming towards us.

We flew out of Oslo as scheduled at 2.15 p.m. Once we were up in the air, Sue and I chatted to each other as the afternoon wore on. We especially enjoyed talking about a trip whenever it came to its end. We liked to sum things up and perhaps say for the first time how we'd really felt about some aspect of it. We talked about where we'd gone, who we'd met, what we'd done, some of the funny times we'd had and what we thought about various parts of the trip. While things were still fresh in our minds, we made a rough list of what we thought were the highlights. Then we both sat back and left each other to our own thoughts again.

Our highlights included the glaciers – so many in that one area in the Svalbard. Seven, with jagged mountain peaks behind them. And the three polar bears, which we wished we could've got closer to, were high on the list.

While we were talking, I realised that, in fact, we'd seen very little wildlife on the trip. The only animals we'd seen on the whole trip were Sue's cat, Carolyn's reindeer and two of the three polar bears. In the far north of the Arctic, the polar bears were the only wildlife we'd seen. This was very different from Antarctica, with its incredible variety and quantity of wildlife. We saw thousands of penguins on that trip to the far south.

However, the polar circle boats on this trip were much better for me than the Zodiacs in Antarctica. The number of landings I'd been able to do really surprised me. The first landing at Magdalenefjord was the hardest and probably the best way to start because it didn't seem very hard at all at the time. It had been a pleasure to visit so many little places along the way.

The beauty of the fjords was more than either of us had expected, with their steep rock faces and waterfalls everywhere.

We thought the Norwegians were friendly people and just about everyone we met spoke English well. But we also agreed that the local tourist advice was not always right. I thought that sometimes you just have to work it out as you go. A good example of this was when we were waiting for a tram for people with disabilities – a tram that didn't exist!

Although it had rained most of the time when we weren't on the cruise, we'd managed with our wet weather gear. We'd just become used to going out wearing all that gear, and then the rain didn't matter. Sometimes, you've got to be out in the rain when you're travelling, even though we'd never do that at home.

We certainly agreed about how useful Raina's advice had been, especially about Vinmonopolet. The European wines were excellent and so much cheaper than in Australia.

By evening, my mind was drifting along as I looked out of the window into the dark sky. Suddenly, I saw a large rectangle of lights on the ground. It looked like a walled city of low-rise buildings in pale earthy colours. I looked at the map on the video screen in front of me. We were flying over Kabul in Afghanistan. My eyes widened, blinked and looked again. Yes, the map was labelled 'Kabul' in the middle of the flight path, and 'Afghanistan' was written beside it.

The big rectangle of lights looked as though it was made by lights on the tops of high walls. The bright individual lights merged to form lines around the perimeter. There were more lights inside, but they were less intense.

In my mind, I had some images of Kabul from the television news and documentaries. I'd also read the book *The Little Coffee Shop of Kabul*. From that high up, the place looked a little like how I'd imagined it might look, only bigger. Unfortunately, I didn't have my iPhone or camera nearby to take a photo. They were both packed in the cabin bag stored above us. The image however, was firmly planted in my brain.

I was very surprised to be flying over a war zone. I didn't recall seeing any flight paths that showed travel over Afghanistan, but we were on one. Australia was involved in the 'war on terror' that began in 2001 after the 11 September attacks on the World Trade Center towers in New York. The war was still on then in September 2011, ten years later.

We landed a few hours later in Bangkok, with five hours to spare between flights. We were last off the aircraft as usual and an attendant with a wheelchair was waiting for me. The attendant led us through the terminal to a special assistance lounge. He registered our presence at the counter and then asked us to wait in the lounge until someone came back to collect us.

He left with the wheelchair. It was in the early hours of the morning and we thought we'd put our heads back and have a sleep. I did some leg stretching and exercises first. There were other people sitting in chairs and nodding off too. Some were old and some were middle-aged. One elderly woman wore a sari. No one seemed to care about me doing some leg exercises.

The staff at the lounge reception desk disappeared out the back, and we could hear them chatting. I slept for about an hour. I woke thinking that I might go wandering around the airport and look at the shops. I couldn't see much from the doorway to the lounge. But I had no wheelchair and I needed one for Sue to take me when she woke.

Sue woke soon too and asked at reception if we could have a wheelchair. They said they were all in use and when it was time to go someone would come to get us. I tried to explain that I wanted to go for a look around and leave the small lounge area. The plane was not going to leave for hours yet.

'You can't leave. You have to stay here.' The lounge wasn't in a security area, it was just a room off a corridor. They didn't know what saying that to me meant. It was like a red flag to a bull! I hate being told what to do if I can't see a good reason for it.

This was the third time that sort of thing had happened to me. I should have learned by now to never give up a wheelchair at an airport unless I was getting on a plane. I found it so frustrating. I liked being independent. It was frustrating enough to have to get Sue to push me. But she'd enjoy a walk with me, I thought, instead of being stuck in the lounge or wandering off on her own.

The first time it happened was in 2007, at London Heathrow. We were transferring flights in London after arriving from Paris on the way to Honolulu. The attendant, who met me at the aircraft door on landing, took me in a wheelchair to a bus to change airport terminals. I got out of the wheelchair in the bus and sat in a seat. When the bus arrived at the next terminal, there was no wheelchair to meet me. I got off with my walking stick and holding on to Sue's arm. I couldn't walk very far at all at the time, only about ten metres.

A woman offering disability assistance was leaning on what looked like a tiny lectern. She waved me to come over to her. I was outside on the footpath about to enter the terminal building. It was quite a long way to walk. I looked around for a wheelchair. There was none to be seen, even though I'd booked one.

I walked over to the woman with some difficulty. I thought *she* could have walked over to *me*! There was no one else waiting for assistance. She spoke to me roughly and told me to walk to the special assistance centre, pointing into the distance. She seemed very unpleasant and irritated. I couldn't see where she was pointing. It wasn't within eyesight. I said, 'I can't walk that far.' I felt upset and belittled.

Unhappy that she had to move, the woman said, 'Oh, I'll get a wheelchair, then,' and walked away. I waited, standing, leaning on my stick and Sue's arm. When the woman eventually came back, I just about fell into the wheelchair. I was exhausted.

The woman 'assisting' wheeled me through security, where I had to take off my shoes. 'Can you walk through the security gate?' asked the security guard.

'Not on my own. I could, maybe, if I used someone's arm and had my walking stick. I can't walk without help.'

'That's not allowed… Oh, all right, then, stay in the wheelchair' said the security guard. The woman said nothing. She wheeled me around the security gate. The guard called for a female security guard to come and pat me down. A woman came over and patted and checked me. 'Arms up. Just checking.'

'Okay.'

The woman wheeled me away after the pat-down. Sue put our bags and my stick through security and collected them on the other side of the scanner. Sue had to dash to catch up with us, as the woman and I were well away from the security area by then. She seemed really annoyed that she had to wheel me. Finally, we went into a small lounge area with about six seats in it. Already waiting there was a woman with only one leg, another woman who seemed to be blind and one or two others.

We checked in at the reception desk and the woman left, taking the wheelchair with her. The reception staff told us to wait until they called us. After some time, we noticed that the time to board was about fifteen minutes away. Sue went up to reception and told the people sitting there that I'd need a wheelchair to get to the plane. There were two staff members there, and they both wore matching outfits that looked like nurse uniforms.

'It's all organised,' said one of them. 'Just wait until you're called.' Time passed and soon it was two minutes from boarding time. We looked at the boarding gate number on our tickets. Sue went for a walk. When she came back she said, 'That gate is a long way away. We'll never make it if we don't leave soon.'

Sue went back to reception to try to get some action but they didn't seem interested. Soon, a man in an electric people-mover came along, driving very fast. He stopped suddenly and jumped out saying, 'Everyone on!'

The reception staff gave everyone a nod to climb on board the vehicle. Sue raced out and spoke with the man. 'Will this take my friend to the aircraft door? She can't walk from the gate. She needs a wheelchair.' The man asked for my boarding pass. Sue showed it to him.

'There must be some mistake,' he said. 'Quick, can you help her on? I'll call for a wheelchair to be at the gate.' Everyone else struggled on to the vehicle. I didn't notice how the woman with one leg managed, or the blind woman. Once we were all on, the man took off, driving quickly. He phoned someone. 'This shouldn't have happened,' he said.

We finally arrived at our gate, which was a good ten to fifteen minutes away even on this fast electric vehicle. A wheelchair was waiting outside the passageway to the air bridge. I got off the electric car and into the wheelchair. The driver left with everyone else on board to go somewhere else.

We were the last people to board the plane and we were so pleased to see pleasant, smiling airline staff offering us warm moist towels. We made it, but what an effort it was!

I'll always remember that event. It was very unpleasant. I was upset and should have written a letter of complaint. But I didn't.

Back then, in 2007, my MS was worse than it is now. It was hard for me to do much walking at all four years ago. The Tysabri infusions I've been receiving since then have meant that my MS has improved, especially my mobility. Also, since that time, I've became more experienced in using a wheelchair at airports. Thankfully, my experiences have been more positive than negative.

One of the big advantages of wheelchair assistance, especially at international airports, is that someone will meet us and take us to where we have to go. That way is usually the fastest. The aircraft attendants really are the best people to take us to the next boarding gate. It's especially helpful if it's a long way away, or involves catching a train or bus, such as at large airports like Singapore's Changi. Going through customs and immigration is faster too. There are no queues at the wheelchair-assistance desks or the 'Staff Only' ones. The staff member usually stays with me or comes back when they say they will. Most of the time, they leave me in a wheelchair too, in case I want to use it. In reality, it's Sue's job or someone else's to wheel me, because I've never come across an airport wheelchair (international or domestic) that I can operate myself. There are no handrims to allow a person to propel the wheels themselves.

In Bangkok, there I was again in a special assistance area with no wheelchair. 'Why don't you go for a walk without me?' I said to Sue. 'I'll rest here, do some reading.'

'I'll see if I come across a wheelchair,' said Sue.

'Okay.'

Sue was back in five minutes with a wheelchair. The two reception staff members were still out the back. I got in the wheelchair and we went out for a walk.

There wasn't much to see, just the usual duty-free goods. I did look at the whisky, though. It always amazes me that I can never find one that I've tried somewhere else and liked, or one that I've read about that's supposed to be very good. I forget the names most of the time. So I didn't buy any.

I looked at the techno things but, as usual, didn't end up buying anything there either. Sue tried a few perfumes. With not much else to do, we went back to the lounge. No one had missed us.

A little later, after some more exercises and a toilet visit (there was one in the lounge area), someone with a wheelchair came to collect me. There was plenty of time to spare. I boarded the plane without any trouble.

Once in the air, the crew served a meal and Sue and I both asked for a glass of wine to go with it. I thought, who cares about what time it was and whether it was the 'right' time for a drink or not! I dozed happily off to sleep afterwards, with wonderful memories and another map brewing in my mind – a map of our trip with our flights added. (Photo 3.8.2)

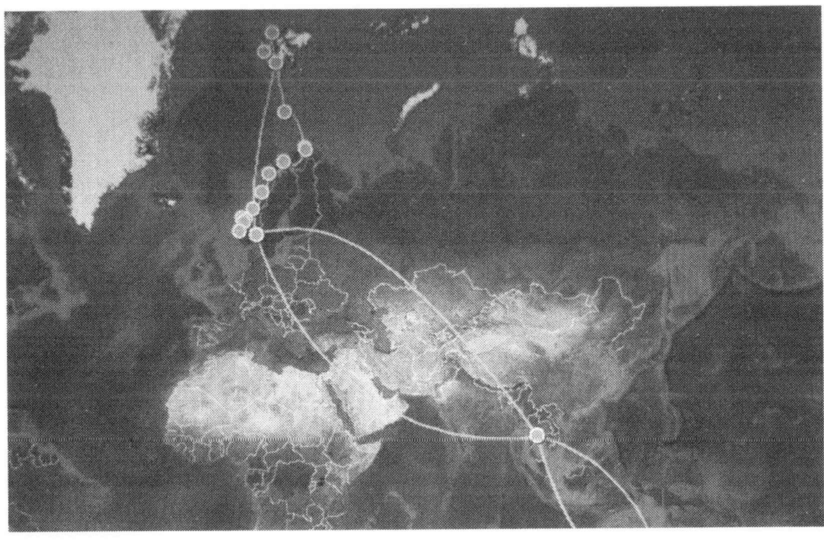

Photo 3.8.2 Map of the trip and our flights
Image credit: Google Maps and Travellerspoint

We landed in Melbourne on Sunday, 25 September, at exactly 8 p.m. An attendant with a wheelchair was at the aircraft door and we sailed through immigration. The scooter and our bag arrived safely off the plane. I rode through customs with nothing to declare.

We caught a taxi home, one of Alan's pre-arranged ones. It was late when we arrived home and it was time for some sleep and rest.

I was feeling a little zonked, but I knew I could switch off at home. That felt good. We were safely back and in plenty of time for my next Tysabri infusion in three days' time.

Things on the list could wait.

PART FOUR:

IN THE END

CHAPTER 1

AFTER THE TRIP

'Don't spill it all out! Keep a bit back. Don't tell it all at once,' Sue berated me. I'd just finished telling someone in the car park about our trip. 'If they want to know more, they'll ask. Leave a bit more to tell.' Sue didn't like playing all her cards at once. Even when she was asked if she'd played golf or squash in the past she'd just say, 'Oh, a little bit.'

I was usually very excited about my trips and keen to tell people everything. Sometimes, it probably *was* too much information. Mum loved hearing a lot of the detail, though. So the next day, when I was thinking again about Myrdal Station – getting down and across those tracks – I couldn't wait to ring her again. I'd already rung to tell her we'd arrived home safely but I didn't go into any detail about the trip.

As I was telling Mum the story about Myrdal, I could feel her listening intently. Every now and then she said, 'Gawd, love, go on,' and 'God help us, love.' Then, in the middle of the story, something sparked off a memory in Mum's mind about a trip she'd taken in the past. That often happened when we were talking about travelling, and she had to tell me straight away. Before she forgot. But she'd never really forgotten because it usually wasn't the first time I'd heard the story! We finished the phone call with her saying, 'I'm really looking forward to seeing the photos when they're ready. Thank you, love, thank you.'

While I was on the phone, Sue had been unpacking and sorting clothes to wash. 'How was Noel?'

'She was good. She loved hearing about us getting over the tracks. I'll have to get on and do those photos too.'

With the unpacking almost done, Sue asked, 'Where do you want me to put these receipts? You'll tell me how much we spent on the trip when you work it out, won't you?'

'Yes, sure. On my desk, please. Just give me a day or so.'

With all the information in those receipts, I included our total costs in the original travel table. I showed Sue the 'Travel Table with $' (Appendix 2). Most of the costs for the Norway and Arctic trip were there. Then I filed it away.

Carolyn soon heard from me too. She was keen to hear how I'd managed and what we'd seen. She also said she was looking forward to seeing the photos. It was time to sort them out.

There were about two thousand photos. I loaded them up on to my computer soon after I arrived home and also made a copy on my external hard drive. I usually made what I called a 'show' – a travel story in photos – within the first month of arriving home from a significant trip. It was time to do just that.

I enjoyed looking at all my photos – selecting the good ones and the ones I needed to make a story – and putting them into a show. I put them into a file named simply 'SHOW of Norway and the Arctic'. Putting the first word in upper case made it stand out in my list of photo files.

But before sharing it with others I wanted to look at it myself on the television screen and remember the trip as one journey. It was also a good final check for any errors. I wanted to watch it with Sue, so I saved the slideshow on to a DVD. That was the best way I knew to look at the photos on a large-screen TV. A DVD was also good because I could file it away in a place that I could quickly and easily get to whenever I wanted to watch it again.

I tried to put the photos together in a way that took me back, as well as showed others for the first time what it had been like. I usually tried to limit the show to about 250 to 300 photos. When the slideshow went at five seconds a frame, this meant it would take just below thirty minutes to run. I thought that was enough. People might drop off to sleep if it went too long!

As I was putting the show of Norway and the Arctic together, I realised that my photos had drastically changed character. They weren't the usual kind of travel photo I'd taken in the past. To start with, there were pictures of things I'd never photographed before: toilet facilities, bathrooms and wheelchair-accessible routes. I'd also taken more photos of motor vehicles than I ever had before – their boots, not their fronts.

That all meant that I had to think differently about what I'd taken, what I was looking at and also about which ones to put in a slideshow for other people.

My usual travel photos were mostly picturesque scenes, landscapes with only a few shots of the people we'd met along the way. I rarely had one taken of myself in front of a significant spot. In general, people were missing. But in the photos of Norway and the Arctic, there were people there as well as those other odd things. Some photos of people were taken long before I'd got to know them. Their presence in the early photos was unintended.

Looking at the photos reminded me that I'd met some very nice people, including some that I thought might become good friends. I enjoyed talking with just about everyone, and I learned so much from some of them.

I could see new things in my photos that were taken as if they were of enormous significance. They included bumpy footpaths where the drains went across them rather than underneath, the gaps at station platforms, power points and gravel sides on roads. Then there were photos of ramps, steps and lifts to get on and off all the forms of transport that I went on. But there was an incredible amount of them. I must have had someone or something in mind when I took them.

The motor vehicles that featured in my photos were not the spunky, sporty vehicles I used to look at many years ago. The vehicle photos were of small vans or station wagons where there was plenty of room for transporting a scooter and other mobility aids. A lot of the vehicles were ones I hadn't seen in Australia. There seemed to be a greater choice in Europe, and I was ripe for looking around in case there was something better than our Golf wagon.

All that made me really think about what I took travel photos of and why. It's probably my science and medical backgrounds that make me ask 'why' a lot. Even before university, my schooling with the most famous scientist in Australia, Professor Harry Messel, with his textbooks and flamboyant television show *Why Is it So?* helped to make me question things.

I suppose I take photos mainly for my own pleasure, but I also like to show them to other people who are interested. Some photos of places were spectacular, such as Magdalenefjord. Others could be useful for people with disabilities planning a trip to the same region perhaps. I had friends in wheelchairs and I liked to show them new things that I'd noticed while I was away.

Photos sometimes said things that words couldn't, like John Brack's paintings. Sometimes photos could speak words and I'd found they could help me write my stories for *DiVine*.

The photo show that I made was a real mix in the end. I organised three hundred trip photos in order and loaded them up on to a web page with Picasa. I sent a link to family and friends. That included my brothers, Carolyn, Robin, Dimitrios, Jan in Tasmania and Jan in Canberra. I also sent a link to Thilli and Anni. I made an extra DVD of the photo show for Mum and posted it to her. Mum always loved looking at my photos. She was probably my biggest fan.

Mum was a good photographer and loved the whole photography scene as a passionate hobby. She'd told me of the time in her teenage years when she'd had her own darkroom under the house to develop her still photos. That was fairly adventurous, I thought, for the 1940s. Mum also bought a movie camera when I was about two or three years old. She had reels of film spools that had changed format from standard 8 to Super 8 as we grew older. Family events, special occasions, ordinary times and holidays were all captured and shown to us on projectors that saw many changes too.

My friend Jan in Tasmania was a good photographer too. She used a very nice Canon digital SLR camera with great skill. It had always amazed me that our photos of the same thing would turn out so differently. Jan would move to a slightly different place to take her photo and she'd take it from a totally different perspective. Her photos always looked better than mine. I loved looking at them.

Jan said she enjoyed looking at my travel photos, but it didn't ever seem to take her very long!

I talked to friends and family (and locals in the car park!) about the trip and tried to tailor the length and detail of what I had to say to each person. But sometimes, I just blurted it all out. As I was telling people, I realised that some of what I was saying was quite different to my other trips. It wasn't just the photos that had changed, there were other things as well.

On the trip, I ended up doing so many new things. I used so many different forms of transport, many for the first time. They included aircraft with no lifters; fast trains, old trains and light rail with different steps and gaps; ferries of various sizes, all with ramps; a cruise ship with ramps and a lift; a motorised dinghy with steps; buses, with and without lower luggage storage for the scooter; trams; cable cars; a funicular; and a familiar station wagon.

Sometimes I didn't know exactly what was going to happen, but I'd learned that was okay. Whatever challenges came up, I'd just deal with them. Besides, no matter how much research I thought I'd done, it was no substitute for being there, seeing the situation for myself and just handling it! I could do more things than I'd realised.

We only used a taxi once – up that steep hill in Ålesund. Sue was right, the public transport options were better. I saw more and felt more 'in the place'.

Sue and I had managed the whole trip on our own. We'd needed some help along the way, but that was no problem. People around us had jumped in and helped. My MS wasn't a problem, and the scooter remained intact and travelled well.

My yellow Luggie scooter is the easiest mobility device I've travelled with yet. It was a big success. The international air flights were the easiest. Those airlines seemed to be less worried about my scooter and its lithium battery than the ones in Australia were. Perhaps they were more experienced, or perhaps they had larger aircraft and it didn't matter as much. They usually had air bridges for international flights, and that made it easier as well. There were never any problems with the scooter on the trip.

In fact, I couldn't have done what I did without the yellow scooter – my chariot! Using it with so much success gave me a huge amount of confidence. I'd definitely needed Sue's help, of course, and she'd also become more confident about what we could do together.

It was good speaking about the trip to others, and putting what it was like into words. Some people were more interested in listening than others. Mum and Carolyn liked a bit more detail.

I wasn't surprised when Mum rang one day to say, 'I've seen your photos, thank you. I was able to get the disc to work on the machine. I sat down with a nice cup of coffee, followed those directions you'd written down and saw them all at one time. Wonderful! I liked the one with the… It reminded me of… And… Oh, and I've heard a lot about the new MONA (Museum of Old and New Art) museum in Tasmania. It sounds quite something – lots of tricky things in it. I think it'd be good to see. It gets cold down there soon, doesn't it?'

'Yes, I've heard about the MONA too.' I love Tasmania, but it does get cold. 'Why not come down to Melbourne while it's warm and we'll go from here? Will you be all right flying on your own?'

'That'd be lovely, love. My back's a lot better now with the pills. It'd be nice to spend a few days in Melbourne with you first.'

We were all soon down in Hobart. The scooter travelled well again, Mum travelled well and I scootered around inside the MONA without any problems at all. The collection of art there was extraordinary. I'm speechless when it comes to trying to explain it.

Being in Hobart was also good because I could catch up with Jan. A group of us, including Mum, went out to a nice restaurant in North Hobart for dinner one night.

'How was the trip?' Jan asked after we'd all sat down.

I told her the Myrdal story.

'That's a good story. You should write that up.'

'Then there was the wheelchair-friendly – I don't think! – cable-car excursion in Tromsø, and the lifts in Oslo …' I went on.

'So many things have happened to you while you've been travelling. People would be interested in hearing about them.' Jan had definitely enjoyed hearing about my travel adventures with my wheelchair in the past, and she seemed even more interested in my scooter stories.

'Do you really think so? Thank you for saying that.'

'Some people might benefit from it and learn too. You should write it all down. And, really, all of that last trip would be good to write about.'

'Okay, I'll think about it.' And, after another half-glass of wine, I did start to think seriously about writing up my trip.

Back in Melbourne, I thought about two really important things. I thought a lot more about the trip and what I might write about it, and I also started to think about our next trip. There's a big permanent area in my brain specifically reserved for travel. That area was always receiving information and ideas. Then a little spot would burst out from the ideas patch one day with a place that I wanted to visit in some foreign country. I needed to have another trip lined up, all the time, to look forward to.

As soon as I started to plan our next trip to Bavaria in Germany and Verona in Italy, I could tell that something was different. Straight away, I could see that my whole approach to planning had completely changed.

I knew I didn't have to plan that next trip so meticulously. My obsession with fine detail wasn't required any more. I knew how capable my scooter was, and I'd learned what I could manage on my own and what Sue and I could manage together. And that seemed to be just about anything! My confidence had skyrocketed.

My view of other things had changed too. I always disagreed with the saying, 'It's the journey, not the destination that counts.' I was always more interested in the destination. That was the whole point, wasn't it? Being where you wanted to go? It was the same feeling I'd had during that Chekov play – for goodness' sake, just go! Just do it. In our last trip, I thought one of the destinations was the Nutshell. Doing at least the kernel was my absolute minimum. I wanted to just get there and do it!

But there were so many more things to the trip than just that tiny Nutshell part of it. And, at one stage, I'd even been thinking of not finishing what I'd planned to do for so long, of not going out in the rain to the famous fjord. Then the penny dropped for me yet again – the Nutshell was part of the journey, not the destination. It was the journey that really mattered after all.

The kernel in the Nutshell was only a side trip lasting less than a day, yet the whole experience – every bit of the Artic and Norway trip – changed my approach to travel and probably to many aspects of everyday living as well.

I was really struck by this business when I went to an exhibition at the State Library of Victoria in Melbourne some time after the trip. It was an exhibition of ancient Persian manuscripts and I learned about the Sufi poets and their writing. I'd never heard of them. They wrote hundreds of years ago, about an approach to life that was different to that of anywhere else in the world at the time. It was mystical and spiritual, and involved that concept of living in the moment, which dates even further back than that time. The journey along the way was the real treasure. That was the meaning of life, according to the Sufi poets.

It was wonderful to learn that. I love learning new things and I also love reading. I read all kinds of things, both light and heavy. The brain – and my brain with its lesions – was particularly interesting to me. Not just what it thought about journeys and destinations, but also why other things had ended up happening to me and to everyone else. I've read quite a few neurological articles and they've mostly been related to some aspect of MS. But there have been other studies, neuroscience ones, that I've found interesting as well.

One of the most interesting ones I'd read since coming back from the trip was an article about 'unexpected rewards'. It was a neuroscience article published in the journal *Nature Neuroscience* and written by Kalyani Narasimhan. In it, I read that:

> Animals (including humans) ... change their behavior based on the possible rewards they receive. When the rewards are different than predicted, there are long-term changes in behavior, but when rewarded exactly as predicted, we do not change our behavior.

I related to that. I understood. I was rewarded many times over when I didn't expect it while doing the Arctic and Norway trip. And my behaviour had already changed – and I could see it changing even more as I started to plan the next trip. I was thinking of taking more chances and not chasing the same level of detail as before. I didn't need to know everything any more, and I didn't need to ask questions or try to find out as much as possible. I was leaving more in the 'unknown' basket.

Something else that I'd learned to stop doing was Googling everything. It was a real joy to sometimes come across things and be surprised, to find something out for myself.

Another interesting neuroscience article I read was published in the *Journal of Neuroscience* and was about MRI brain scans. It wasn't a study of MS lesions, but rather of the brain's 'pleasure spots'. In the study, the brain's pleasure centres 'lit up' on MRI scans when the subject experienced unpredicted pleasant experiences. It was reported that according to the authors of the study, this indicated that:

> ...the brain finds unexpected pleasure more rewarding than expected ones, and it may have little to do with what people say they like.

That was fascinating research, I thought.

And I went on to think that perhaps one good reason why I and so many others experience a special feeling from travel could be because it was a big supplier of unpredictable pleasant experiences, and that really turned the brain's pleasure spots on! Travel can be addictive and now I understand why.

I want to keep travelling for as long as I can. Travelling and looking for opportunities to do it will continue to be desires that drive me, I'm sure. It gives me so much enjoyment and so many rewards.

One final reason I enjoyed the Artic and Norway trip so much could have been because of yet another one of my mother's many sayings. When she heard about any challenge I faced, big or small, she'd say, 'Give it your best shot, lovey. Give it a go.' That was really important to her. Even if I failed, she'd say, 'At least you gave it a go.' And that probably summed up how she lived her life – in a nutshell.

I think she instilled that attitude in me too. I gave it a go. I gave it my best shot. I realised that was important to me too. The trip – the journey *and* the destination – was full of unexpected rewards. My brain's pleasure spots were all well and truly lit up, turned on and left wanting more. On to the next trip now!

THE END of this one

POSTSCRIPT

When I was nearly at the end of writing this book, my mother died suddenly of cardiovascular problems. Jan in Tasmania was dying of ovarian cancer. My mother talked of travelling right until the end. Jan continued to encourage me and she was able to read a few chapters in her last months. She died three months after Mum did.

I'm grateful to Sue because, without her, I couldn't have done what I did on the trip. We continue to travel with my scooter and returned to the Arctic to visit Iceland.

After a recent trip to Japan, I was asked to return and give a talk to people with disabilities – to 'give them a dream' and show them that travelling is still possible even if you have mobility problems. I gave the talk and I hope this book encourages people with any mobility problem to get and about with their aids.

My MS remains stable on Tysabri and I hope that, with my story of MS and this trip, as Jan said, 'Some people might benefit from it.'

I keep travelling because I love it and because I want to see as much as I can while I can. I'm going to keep giving it a go and my best shot.

APPENDIX 1
PACKING LIST
NORWAY & THE ARCTIC, SEPTEMBER 2011

<u>Gloves</u>
- Gortex-MC
- Ac/Poly/El-SW (of C)

<u>Beanie</u>
- Red-MC

w red & white band
- Black-SW (of C)

w purple band

<u>Warm Thermal Long Underwear</u>
- Black Pants -MC
  -SW
- Black Top -MC
  -SW

<u>Neck Warmers</u>
- MC
- SW

<u>Pants</u>
- MC -Beige (wear)
  -Black
  -Blue check
  -Black Track Pants (warm polartec)
- SW -Lgt Grey (wear)
  -Good Black
  -black ExOfficio
  -?take trackpants

<u>Wet Weather Pants</u>
- MC -of BW
- SW -from golf (to wash)

<u>Nighties</u>
- Pale Blue -MC
- Navy -SW

<u>Good Tops</u>
- Green Black White Shirt
  -SW
- Autumn Leaves Shirt
  -MC
- Blue Hedrena - SW (carry on)
- Blue Black Animal Stripes
  -MC
- Purple Dot Collared Jumper
  -SW

<u>Scarves</u>
- Grey Black -MC (wear)
- Red Black Animal-MC
- Leopard Tiger Animal-SW

<u>Shoes</u>
- Black w Stitching-MC
- Maroon Red-MC (wear)

- First Aid Kit
- Psyllium 200gm

<u>BACKPAK</u>

<u>Chargers</u>
- Luggie
- Nikon camera
- Power adaptors
- Video camera
- Mobile phone

-Poncho
-Blow up pillow ?
-Aircraft set (toothb,mask,earplug)
-Pills, Drs letters

<u>Casual Tops</u>
- Black T Shirt (Ed B)-MC (wear)
- Hot Pink-SW
- Teal Blue w zip-SW
- Black Long Sleeve Sussan-SW
- Purple Strip Collar-SW
- Purple Long Sleeves –MC
- Maroon Polartec-MC

So far - SW (7) MC(6)
- Kelvin Klein Grey w Collar-MC

<u>Bras</u>
- MC x 2 (wear 1, 1 in wash)
- SW x 2 (wear 1, 1 to go in)

<u>Underpants</u>
- MC -1 beige (wear) ExO
  -2 black ExO
- SW -1 black
  -2 cotton (wear 1)

<u>Sox</u>
- MC -Bed sox
  -Blue thick cotton w pattern
  -Black wool (wear)
  -Navy wool
- SW-Black bamboo
  -Black thin cotton
  -Black Bonds (wear)
  -Thick yellow

<u>Coats</u>
- Black Gortex -MC (of C)
- Black Snowgum –SW (of M)
- Rainjackets x 2

- Aqium hand gel
- Aeroguard roll-on insect repel
- Clothes washing/Line }
Powder/sewing } bag

Weight of bag at airport = 18kg

APPENDIX 2
TRAVEL TABLE WITH $
NORWAY & THE ARCTIC, SEPTEMBER 2011

Day	Date Sept	Day	Travel Transport	Location	Accommodation	Booked	Paid/Ref
1	1	Thurs	Fly	Depart Melb 3pm for Oslo	On plane Thai Airways	√ (flight)	√ YES $4,124 return
2	2	Fri	Stay	Arrive Oslo 0725 am	Frogner House Apartments Arbinsgate 3 Oslo	√ (accom)	√ YES $920.70 five nites Visa Hotels.com
3	3	Sat	Stay	Oslo	Frogner House Apartments Oslo	√ (accom)	YES "
4	4	Sun	Stay	Oslo	Frogner House Apartments Oslo	√ (accom)	YES "
5	5	Mon	Stay	Oslo	Frogner House Apartments Oslo	√ (accom)	YES "
6	6	Tues	Stay	Oslo	Frogner House Apartments Oslo	√ (accom)	YES "
7	7	Weds	Fly to Cruise trip day 1	Fly Oslo to Longyearbyen	Longyearbyen Rad Blu Polar Hotel	√ cruise trip	√ YES cruise trip $11,206
8	8	Thurs	Board Ship Cruise day 2	Longyearbyen and Barentsburg	Ship MS Fram	√ cruise trip	"
9	9	Fri	Cruise day 3	Magdalenefjord and Moffen	Ship MS Fram	"	"
10	10	Sat	Cruise day 4	Ny Alesund	Ship MS Fram	"	"
11	11	Sun	Cruise day 5	Bjornoya (Bear Island)	Ship MS Fram	"	"
12	12	Mon	Cruise day 6	Honningsvag	Ship MS Fram	"	"
13	13	Tues	Cruise day 7	Tromso	Ship MS Fram	"	"
14	14	Weds	Cruise day 8	Trollfjord and Henningsvaer	Ship MS Fram	"	"
15	15	Thurs	Cruise day 9	Alstahaug and Vega	Ship MS Fram	"	"
16	16	Fri	Cruise d 10	Brekstad	Ship MS Fram	"	"
17	17	Sat	Cruise d 11	Alesund and Geiranger	Ship MS Fram	"	"
18	18	Sun	Cruise d 12	Olden, Nordfjord	Ship MS Fram	"	"
19	19	Mon	Cruise d 13 end Stay	Bergen	Augustin Hotel	√ accomm	NO-pay there fjord pass $660 3 nites
20	20	Tues	Stay	Bergen	Augustin Hotel	"	NO-pay there fjord pass
21	21	Weds	Stay	Bergen	Augustin Hotel	"	NO-pay there fjord pass
22	22	Thurs	Train & stay	Flam	Flamsbrygga Hotel	√ accomm ferry yet	NO-pay there fjord pass $240
			Trains		Total NSB trains		√ YES Trains $534
23	23	Fri	Train & stay	Oslo	Thon Hotel Opera	√ accomm	√ YES $225.50 Visa Hotels.com
24	24	Sat	Fly	Dep Oslo 2.15 pm	Plane Thai Air		Paid above
25	25	Sun	Fly	Arrive Melb 8pm	Home		

All costs known before leaving for two people amounted to $17,910.20. Then the additional amounts for short train trips, ferry trips, excursions, meals and miscellane-ous came to about another $1,600 for two. So it was about $19,510 all up for two or $9,755 each.

APPENDIX 3
CRUISE STOPS TABLE

Place Port	Trip Day No.	Cruise Day No.	Spitsbergen Landing No.	Mainland Landing No.	Extra Excur-sions
Longyear-byen	7	1	1		
Barentsburg	8	1	2		
Magda-lenefjord	9	2	3		
Moffen	9		At sea		
Ny-Ålesund	10	3	4		
Bear Island at sea	11	4	5		
Honningsvåg	12	5		1	Nord-kapp by bus
Tromsø	13	6		2	Cable car by bus
Svolvær and Henningsvær	14	7		3	
Alstahaug and Vega	15	8		4 and 5	
Brekstad	16	9		6	
Ålesund and Geiranger	17	10		7 and 8	Gei-ranger pano-rama by bus
Olden Nordfjordeid	18	11		9 and 10	
Bergen	19	12		11	

Printed in Australia
AUOC02n2205221116
280764AU00003B/3/P

9 781925 442472